A Guide to the MRCP
Part 2 Written Paper

A Guide to the MRCP
Part 2 Written Paper

Anthony N. Warrens BSc, BM, BCh, MRCP (UK)
MRC Clinician Scientist Fellow and Honorary Senior Registrar, Renal Unit,
Royal Postgraduate Medical School, Hammersmith Hospital, London, UK

Stephen H. Powis BSc, BM, BCh, MRCP (UK)
MRC Clinician Scientist Fellow and Honorary Senior Registrar, Renal Unit,
United Medical and Dental School, Guy's Hospital, London, UK

Malcolm Persey MA, MB, BS, MRCP (UK)
Medical Registrar, Northwick Park Hospital, London, UK

and

Alimuddin Zumla PhD, MRCP (UK)
Associate Professor, Center for Infectious Diseases,
University of Texas Health Science Center, Houston, Texas, USA

With additional material from

Shaun McGee
R. Campbell Tait

CHAPMAN & HALL MEDICAL
London · Glasgow · Weinheim · New York · Tokyo · Melbourne · Madras

Published by Chapman & Hall, 2-6 Boundary Row, London SE1 8HN, UK

Chapman & Hall, 2-6 Boundary Row, London SE1 8HN, UK

Blackie Academic & Professional, Wester Cleddens Road, Bishopbriggs, Glasgow G64 2NZ, UK

Chapman & Hall GmbH, Pappelallee 3, 69469 Weinheim, Germany

Chapman & Hall USA, One Penn Plaza, 41st Floor, New York, NY10119, USA

Chapman & Hall Japan, ITP - Japan, Kyowa Building, 3F, 2-2-1 Hirakawacho, Chiyoda-ku, Tokyo 102, Japan

Chapman & Hall Australia, Thomas Nelson Australia, 102 Dodds Street, South Melbourne, Victoria 3205, Australia

Chapman & Hall India, R. Seshadri, 32 Second Main Road, CIT East, Madras 600 035, India

First edition 1994
Reprinted 1994

© 1994 Anthony N. Warrens, Stephen H. Powis, Malcolm Persey and Alimuddin Zumla

Typeset in 10/12pt Palatino by Cotswold Typesetting Ltd, Gloucester
Printed in Great Britain at the University Press, Cambridge

ISBN   0 412 43470 9

A Catalogue record for this book is available from the British Library

Library of Congress Cataloging-in-Publication Data
A Guide to the MRCP part 2 written paper/Anthony N. Warrens....[et al.]; with the additional material from Shaun McGee, R. Campbell Tait.-1st ed.
p.   cm.
Includes index.
ISBN0-412-43470-9
1. Internal medicine-Examinations, questions, etc.I. Warrens, Anthony.
[DNLM:1. Medicine-examination questions. W 18 G9463 1993]
RC58.G835   1993
616'.0076-dc20
DNLM/DLC
for Library of Congress 93-23428 CIP

CONTENTS

FOREWORD

Publishers are convinced that forewords sell books. This book needs no foreword for it will be a smash hit in its own right. The authors have put together a volume which will undoubtedly carry postgraduates through the MRCP and beyond. It is a pleasure to assess its potential, to pit oneself against these authors' quick wits, and moreover it is a joy to read. The authors are born teachers of medicine who have honed their skills on the sharp cutting edge of London hospital registrarmanship where teaching is a daily event. It is to their credit that they have assembled such a mass of facts, which is accurately designed for the examination in mind. This sophisticated data bank is also recommended for other higher examinations in medicine around the world.

Exam-sitting postgraduates must use this book just to make doubly sure that they will pass. It is also recommended for their examiners, who need occasional updates to keep pace with their candidates. But there is an even wider market for this book. In the United States there is an admirable scheme of recertification of doctors which is widely pursued because their practice and livelihood depend on keeping up to date. The Australian College of Physicians is to be congratulated for planning to introduce recertification in 1994. Such a scheme is long overdue in Britain. Our better, more diligent, doctors keep abreast of advances by lectures and conferences. They should also study this book so that they can confidently face any future recertification tests with equanimity.

Dear examination candidate, don't spend any more time on this needless foreword; just go ahead and enjoy this excellent book.

D Geraint James MA, MD, FRCP
Visiting Professor of Medicine
Royal Free Hospital Medical School, London
May, 1993

PREFACE

Why another Membership book? When you pass the Membership there is a feeling that you have now successfully clambered over the final hurdle of the ever more demanding obstacle course put there to torment you by 'The System': O levels, A levels, Finals and then the MRCP. It is sadly true that there are more hurdles round the corner, but those are somehow different. The Membership is the last time they give you a number and you feel part of a herd. From the other side of that hurdle you look back and see colleagues, often contemporaries or people only months your junior. You have learned something about the peculiarities of the jump – where the approach is uneven, how best to launch yourself, etc. There is a natural wish to want to pass on that information. But have we anything to pass on that is not already available in print?

A lot of Membership books essentially present the information available from a standard textbook of medicine and rearrange it in the form of Membership-style questions and answers. Sadly, at this stage knowledge is not enough; there is a technique necessary to answer MRCP questions and this is rarely discussed in books. What we have tried to do in this book is to distill the advice we were given on pre-exam courses and in the bar by more senior colleagues. We have added some of our own experiences and prejudices and then tried to present that information in the context of typical questions and answers. We have tried to make the book as representative as possible across the spectrum of general medicine. However, we have emphasized those areas we feel are least well understood by candidates. In this way we hope we will make the exam less daunting.

We wish you luck – and hope we have helped minimize your need for it.

Anthony N. Warrens
Stephen H. Powis
Malcolm Persey
Alimuddin Zumla

ACKNOWLEDGEMENTS

We have often wondered if authors merely thanked their wives for form's sake, and, we dare say, in some cases they do. But in the case of this book, the active encouragement, support and practical help from our wives has been a major contribution and source of pleasure.

We are grateful also to everyone at Chapman & Hall for their help in producing this book. In particular, Paul Remes who encouraged, bullied and supported us as was appropriate at each stage. Without his help, this book may have been the first Membership book of the twenty-first century. We should also like to thank Jo Dennis and Tausi Seremba for keeping the momentum going to the final whistle.

In an attempt to maximize the value and to minimize the number of errors in this book, we have asked both senior colleagues from various specialities and junior colleagues on the verge of taking the exam to review the material. Their contribution has been invaluable and we should like to record our gratitude to each of them:

Dr A. Ansari	Miss J.M. Heaton	Dr W. Rakowicz
Dr J. Ball	Prof D. Isenberg	Dr B. Ramsey
Dr C. Baynes	Dr G. Llewelyn	Dr W. Rosenberg
Dr E. Beck	Dr A. Lulat	Dr N. J. Simmonds
Dr R. Behrens	Prof K.P.W.J. McAdam	Dr A.K.L. So
Dr J. Chambers	Dr D. McEnirey	Dr S.M. Tighe
Dr P. Chiodini	Dr T. McKay	Dr W.R.C. Weir
Dr E. Choi	Dr S. Makinole	Dr P.R. Wilkinson
Mr J. Conway	Dr P.D. Mason	Dr M.K.B. Whyte
Dr F. Flinter	Dr M. Medlock	Dr P. Wong
Dr M. Friston	Dr P. Nunn	

Finally, we should like to single out two colleagues who have made a major contribution to this book:

Dr Shaun McGee
Department of Radiology
University Hospital of Wales
Cardiff
Wales, UK

Dr Campbell Tait
Department of Haematology
Hope Hospital
Salford
Lancs., UK

HOW TO USE THIS BOOK

It is often said that the second part of the MRCP (UK) entrance examination is the toughest test an aspiring physician must face. Candidates do not need reminding that only about one-third will pass at any one sitting. The aim of this book is to increase the likelihood of success in the written section of the examination.

Candidates fail for two main reasons. Either they lack the degree of knowledge required or their examination technique is poor. The College has no syllabus, so preparation for the examination is difficult. It is hard to know how much should be covered and in what depth. This book contains many examples of questions we think might come up, but we could never hope to cover all possibilities. This is where a good examination technique becomes indispensable.

Knowing all there is to know about medicine does not necessarily guarantee success in the MRCP – although of course it would be a great asset! It is rather like the football manager who knows everything about the game, but fails to study the tactics of the opposite team – he can still be beaten. Likewise, you must have a plan going into examination. It is no good memorizing the contents of numerous textbooks without ever having tried a specimen question. Quite simply, approach the examination as if you were going into battle with the College – not such an inappropriate analogy. You must develop an examination technique which will allow you to make the best use of your knowledge on the day. We have deliberately structured our book to help you achieve this.

The book has three sections which correspond to the three parts of the written examination: Section 1, Case Histories (or 'grey' cases); Section 2, Data Interpretation; Section 3, Pictorial Material. Each section has an introduction discussing examination technique – read this before starting to answer the questions. After this we present a number of papers which you should work your way through, one at a time. Try to work under examination conditions, attempting to answer all the questions in the allocated time before looking at the answers. Paying attention to time is of great importance. You would be well advised to write down your answers otherwise you will tend to credit yourself with an answer that passed through your mind, even if you rejected it. If you have written evidence of your final conclusion, you are likely to come away with a similar impression to the one you will create on the examiners. In addition, writing down answers will get you into the discipline of phrasing answers in their most complete form.

When it comes to sitting the examination, if you are asked for three answers and you write down four, the fourth one will be discarded, even if it is the only one that is right. Take care to play by the College's rules – after all you are applying to join.

When you do look at the answers, you will find detailed descriptions of how to approach the particular kind of question you have been set. Extra information is provided in two types of boxes. In the shaded boxes we present generalized tips on technique. In the unshaded boxes we present information that you may find particularly useful in tackling the examination. (You will find these listed alphabetically at the end of the book for ease of reference, in addition to the more general index.) In subsequent papers, you will encounter similar types of question. If you have read and understood the discussion provided with the first example, then these should become progressively easier to tackle. For example, in the first echocardiogram question, we shall discuss how best to approach an echocardiogram and what diagnoses to expect. At each subsequent echocardiogram question, we shall remind you where to find the full discussion.

Throughout the book, possible answers are listed under the headings 'accepted answers' and 'rejected answers'. Within the list of accepted answers are groups separated by extra wide spaces. Each group will attract progressively fewer marks than the group above it. We have attempted to quantify how inferior each successive group is. This emphasizes the importance of giving as much information as possible in your answer, and of using terms very carefully. The 'rejected answers' include those which you might think would be accurate, but which either disregard an important piece of information with which it would be incompatible, or are too simplistic to be acceptable. This approach will only be applicable to certain questions.

Example:

Accepted answers	*Rejected answers*
Haemolytic crisis due to sickle cell anaemia (100%)	Haemolytic anaemia
Sickle cell anaemia (50%) Sickle cell crisis (50%)	
Haemolytic crisis (25%)	

Comments

The answer required to attract full marks needs to mention both sickle cell anaemia and haemolytic crisis. The word 'crisis' alone gains no more marks than 'sickle cell anaemia' alone as there are other type of crisis in sickle cell disease. Mentioning the underlying cause of the problem, 'sickle cell anaemia', attracts more marks than noting that there is a haemolytic crisis. 'Haemolytic anaemia' alone is inadequate to gain any marks.

This style is based on the Colleges' own model answers book (which we recommend you buy). Clearly, the ranking of answers is open to debate. No one can actually say how the colleges will feel in any given situation. However, in each ranking there is a principle being illustrated.

We have attempted to be as comprehensive as possible, but there will clearly be important gaps. There is also occasional repetition. This is deliberate. Having dealt with a case of Spotty's disease in paper 1 you have no grounds for excluding old Spotty as an explanation for a particularly difficult example in paper 7.

Our list of rejected answers will reflect our own insecurities and ignorance. There will be cases where we do not help you to understand why this man's hemiplegia is not due to his acne.

All we can say is that we have done our best. Please feel free to write to us (c/o Chapman & Hall) with other areas of discussion that you feel should have been included as well as criticism of what is here.

SECTION 1

SECTION 1 – CASE HISTORIES

This section is difficult to prepare for because you really could be asked almost anything. More than ever you are relying on your overall knowledge and experience of general medicine.

Having said that, you can still optimize your chance by employing a logical examination technique. Some case histories can be surprisingly short and the answers straightforward. In these you often either know the answer or you don't. Some cases, however, are truly 'grey', and for examples you are finding difficult, we suggest you adopt the following approach.

- Differentiate the 'hard data' from the 'soft data'. By 'hard data' we mean unequivocal abnormalities: these are usually physical signs or abnormal laboratory results. The history can provide hard data but remember, as in real clinical practice, what the patient says might not be entirely correct and some important information may be withheld. This often has to be regarded as soft data. You may assume that physical signs have been correctly elicited and reported and also that the examiner is not withholding from you a relevant physical sign which you would expect to find on thorough routine examination.
- Next construct a differential diagnosis around a piece of hard data, for example, eosinophilia or hypercalcaemia from the laboratory data, or splenomegaly from the physical examination. Choose the most unusual observation.
- Finally, use the softer data to narrow your differential diagnosis until you reach a diagnosis.

In the papers that follow, we will try to illustrate this technique wherever appropriate.

When you reach the examination, there are certain rules you should stick to, if at all possible. These hold true for all sections of the examination:

- If you are having difficulty with a question, move on and come back to it later. Time is limited and there is nothing more soul destroying than running out of time because you have spent too long on a question you could not do.
- Be precise in what you write. The College can be quite fussy over the way they award marks. Similarly, don't use abbreviations: write chest X-ray or chest radiograph, not CXR.

One final point: just as 'grey cases' can be difficult for candidates, they can also be difficult for authors of books such as this. We cannot always predict exactly which answers or wording would attract the most marks in the eyes of the College. No doubt at times you will disagree with our interpretations but, unfortunately, this is the very essence of the grey case! If you disagree with us every so often, you are very probably right. But if you disagree with us a lot, remember that these questions have been seen by a lot of people before ever coming to print. You have to ask yourself if you have an unreasonable degree of self-confidence. Unfortunately, this is often a cause of failure in the MRCP. Better you should learn the lesson in the privacy of your own room from a book than from the Colleges' examiners. Excuse our forwardness.

Case Histories Paper 1

1.1

A 38-year-old City solicitor was admitted because of rapidly increasing jaundice immediately following her return from holiday in Ibiza. She had been entirely well prior to leaving the UK 2 weeks previously. Five days before her return she began to feel unwell and 2 days later she was first noted to have developed jaundice. She experienced mild epigastric fullness and discomfort, anorexia and nausea. She was now unable to keep any food down and still complained of abdominal fullness.

She had smoked 5–10 cigarettes/day for 20 years and drank three or four glasses of wine on social occasions, on average three times per week, although she had drunk 'rather more' on holiday. She denied intravenous or other drug abuse and had had no recent blood transfusions. She knew of no infectious contacts. She was married and had no other sexual partners.

On examination, she was jaundiced but afebrile. She was slightly drowsy and displayed a minor coarse tremor. There was some evidence of constructional apraxia. There were no stigmata of chronic liver disease. She was mildly tender in the epigastrium but there was no hepatic or splenic enlargement. There was no lymphadenopathy. Her blood pressure was 145/70 mmHg lying and 150/80 mmHg sitting. The rest of the examination was normal.

Her full blood count was normal. The results of further investigations were as follows:

Plasma sodium	132 mmol/l
Plasma potassium	3.9 mmol/l
Plasma urea	24.7 mmol/l
Plasma creatinine	198 μmol/l
Plasma plasma aspartate aminotransferase	554 IU/l *(normal range 4–20)*
Plasma alkaline phosphatase	900 IU/l *(normal range 30–100)*
Hb	12.4 g/dl
Wbc	8.2×10^9/l
Platelets	235×10^9/l
Prothrombin time	34 s (control 14 s)
Partial thromboplastin time	51 s (control 34 s)
Chest X-ray showed no abnormalities	
Plain abdominal radiograph showed no abnormalities	
HBsAg	negative
Urinalysis	no cells, protein, or glucose specific gravity 1.030

What is the diagnosis?

1.2

A 26-year-old intravenous drug abuser was brought as an emergency to casualty by his girl-friend. Four days prior to admission he had developed fever, non-productive cough and generalized muscle aches. Despite being prescribed amoxycillin and erythromycin by his GP he had become worse and was now dyspnoeic. He had recently returned from a visit to Morocco. He drank heavily and smoked 30 cigarettes per day. He and his girlfriend had been treated for syphilis 3 months previously.

On examination he was acutely ill, centrally cyanosed with a temperature of 38.8°C, normotensive and had a pulse of 100/min. He had mild jaundice, oral candidiasis and tattoo marks on his right forearm. There were a few bilateral fine crackles on auscultation of the chest. His venepuncture sites were clean. There was no clinical evidence of deep vein thromboses of the calves.

The results of investigations were as follows:

Hb	12.8 g/dl
Wbc	$12 \times 10^9/l$
ESR	42 mm in first hour
Plasma sodium	136 mmol/l
Plasma potassium	3.5 mmol/l
Plasma urea	5.1 mmol/l
Plasma creatinine	98 μmol/l
Plasma bilirubin	90 μmol/l
Plasma plasma aspartate aminotransferase	56 IU/l (*normal range 4–20*)
Plasma γ-glutamyl transferase	101 IU/l (*normal range 7–33*)
Plasma alkaline phosphatase	306 IU/l (*normal range 30–100*)

ECG: sinus tachycardia
Chest X-ray: fine ground glass shadowing in both upper and mid zones

Arterial blood gases	pH	7.46
(on 30% oxygen)	PaO_2	7.0 kPa
	$PaCO_2$	3.8 kPa
Blood cultures		negative
Cold agglutinins		negative
Urinalysis		no abnormality

(a) What is the likely diagnosis?
(b) Which two investigations would you perform?
(c) Which two treatments would you prescribe?

1.3

A 33-year-old nurse had been an insulin-dependent diabetic since the age of 16. She had managed her diabetes attentively and had remained in good health. She developed a 'flu-like illness while on a strenuous walking holiday in the Lake District. Several days later, she noticed that she had developed shortness of breath on exertion and returned home several days early. However, she became increasingly breathless and was admitted to hospital.

On examination, she was well at rest but became mildly dyspnoeic on minimal exertion. She was apyrexial. She had a few crepitations at her right base but her left hemithorax was clear. She had a pulse of 108/min at rest and a blood pressure of 115/65 mmHg. She had mild ankle oedema and her JVP was raised 4 cm with normal waveform. Urinalysis was normal.

Her chest X-ray showed some shadowing at the right base and a cardiac silhouette at the upper limit of normal. Her ECG showed minor T wave inversion in all the chest leads. On admission, the results of initial investigations were as follows:

Plasma sodium	131 mmol/l
Plasma potassium	3.4 mmol/l
Plasma urea	12.6 mmol/l
Hb	14.4 g/dl
Wbc	7.2×10^9/l
Platelets	335×10^9/l

(a) What is the diagnosis?
(b) What further investigation would be most useful?

1.4

A 30-year-old woman presented to casualty as an emergency, having developed a widespread, symmetrically distributed, macular rash and ulceration of the mucous membranes of the mouth, eyes and vagina. She gave a 3-day history of a sore throat and 'flu-like illness for which she was prescribed amoxycillin by her GP.

Her 6-year-old son had had chickenpox 2 weeks ago. She had never been abroad. She owned a budgie and an Alsatian dog. There was no history of allergies.

On examination, she was acutely ill and distressed with a temperature of 39.2°C but was normotensive. There was conjunctival injection and small beads of pus were seen at the inner canthus. There were painful ulcers in the mouth and in the genital tract. Erythematous macules of varying size were distributed all over the body including the palms and soles of her feet. There were some erythematous lesions and three bullous lesions on her thigh. Urinalysis was normal.

Investigations yielded the following results:

Hb	11.2 g/dl
Wbc	10.8×10^9/l (65% neutrophils)
ESR	36 mm in first hour
Chest X-ray	normal
VDRL	negative
Mycoplasma serology	negative
Throat swab	no growth

(a) What is the diagnosis?
(b) List three possible precipitating agents in this case.

1.5

You are asked to see a 76-year-old-man who has been brought into Casualty by his home help. She told the Casualty receptionist that the patient was 'not quite himself' but gave no further information and left before being seen by a nurse or doctor. You are unable to find another informant. His old notes report several attendances to the rheumatology clinic because of degenerative joint disease.

The patient himself is inattentive and drowsy. He can give you no coherent history. On examination there are no other physical signs. Although he resists neurological examination, there is no obvious focal deficit.

What are the first six investigations you would perform?

1.6

A 19-year-old girl is referred for investigation of headaches. These had started 2 months previously and were worse in the mornings. She had previously been well, having visited her general practitioner previously only for treatment of severe acne. At that time the doctor had also given her contraceptive advice.

Examination showed her to be obese with an unsteady gait and some blurring of the optic disc margins. Her acne was very well controlled.

(a) What do you wish to ask the patient?
(b) What are your first and second diagnostic investigations?
(c) What is the diagnosis, its most important complication, and how would you treat it?

Case Histories Paper 2

2.1

The day after returning from a 6-week holiday to the Philippines, Nepal and India, a 28-year-old doctor developed diarrhoea, abdominal pain and anorexia. He prescribed kaolin and morphine for himself. Ten days later the diarrhoea had become worse producing bloodless, pale, foul-smelling stools. He also had borborygmi, flatulence, anorexia and lethargy and had lost 5 kg in weight. He had taken the recommended course of anti-malarial chemoprophylaxis and had received typhoid, hepatitis B, yellow fever and rabies vaccination as well as human normal immunoglobulin. Whilst in India he had been treated for shigella dysentery with co-trimoxazole.

On examination he looked chronically ill, thin, pale, and fluid depleted. His temperature was 36.8°C. He had pitting of the nails and small patches of psoriasis on the forearm and back. His abdomen had stretch marks and was not distended or tender. The liver and spleen were not palpable. The bowel sounds were increased in frequency and duration. The stools were pale, soft and yellow. Sigmoidoscopy and urinalysis were normal.

Investigations performed revealed the following results:

Hb	12.7 g/dl
Wbc	6.2×10^9/l
Plasma sodium	140 mmol/l
Plasma potassium	4.1 mmol/l
Plasma urea	5.5 mmol/l
Serum albumin	26 g/l
Serum total protein	81 g/l
Plasma aspartate aminotransferase	20 IU/l *(normal range 4–20)*
Plasma alanine aminotransferase	42 IU/l *(normal range 2–17)*
Serum bilirubin	6 μmol/l
Serum immunoglobulins: IgG	14.0 g/l *(normal range 7.2–19.0)*
IgM	1.3 g/l *(normal range 0.5–2.0)*
IgA	6.5 g/l *(normal range 0.8–5.0)*
Blood film	negative for malaria and filaria
Stool culture	no significant bacterial pathogens isolated
72-h faecal fat	140 mmol/l *(normal range 11–18 mmol/l)*

(a) List two possible diagnoses.
(b) Which single investigation is likely to be most informative?

2.2

A 28-year-old American marine presents with fever, red eyes, backache, and swelling and pain in his right knee and left ankle joints. Following a urethral discharge whilst he was in Thailand three weeks previously, he had been treated for gonorrhoea. His mother had severe rheumatoid arthritis and an aunt had diabetes mellitus.

On examination he had a temperature of 38.2°C. The right knee and left ankle joints were tender, hot and swollen with restricted movement. Pressure over the sacroiliac joints and ischial tuberosities caused some pain. He had painful mouth ulcers and brown macules on the sole of his left foot. There was bilateral conjunctivitis. A small bead of discharge was seen at the tip of the urethra. The remainder of the examination was normal.

The results of investigations were as follows:

Hb	14.8 g/dl
Wbc	$14.4 \times 10^9/l$ (69% neutrophils)
ESR	44 mm in first hour
VDRL	negative
Rheumatoid factor	negative
Plasma uric acid	270 μmol/l
	(normal range male: 210–480 μmol/l)
Aspirate of knee effusion:	straw coloured fluid, no organisms seen on microscopy or grown on culture

(a) What is the likely diagnosis?
(b) What are the lesions on the sole of the foot?
(c) List three investigations which would help with diagnosis.

2.3

A 32-year-old renal transplant recipient presents with dyspnoea 6 weeks after transplantation. She had required transplantation after a rapid and irreversible deterioration in renal function due to type I diabetes mellitus. She had had one episode of acute rejection 10 days after trans-plantation which had been reversed with high-dose corticosteroids. She was discharged 3 weeks after transplantation on prednisolone, azathioprine and cyclosporin A with a plasma creatinine of 119 μmol/l. She had failed to present for regular review for 2 weeks before the present assessment.

On examination, she was afebrile and clinically well. Palpation of the graft was unremarkable.

Results of investigations were as follows:

Plasma sodium	144 mmol/l
Plasma potasisum	4.9 mmol/l
Plasma urea	20.2 mmol/l
Plasma creatinine	343 μmol/l

Suggest four diagnostic investigations.

2.4

A 23-year-old male presented to casualty because he had become breathless during the course of the day. He was a non-smoker with no past history of disease.

On examination, he is dyspnoeic on moderate exertion with a respiratory rate of 20/min and a regular pulse of 100/min. His first and second heart sounds are normal, but there is an added systolic click.

(a) What is the diagnosis?
(b) What investigation would you perform to prove this?

2.5

A 26-year-old man was brought to casualty from the local main line station where he had been found drunk, unable to give a history. On examination, he had gross erythema and oedema of his left conjunctiva, was covered in tattoos and smelled of alcohol. The rest of the examination and all initial investigations revealed no further abnormality.

The following morning, he admitted to be under the out-patient care of a psychiatrist on account of his desire to 'scratch the back of his eyeball'. He could not explain why he wanted to do this. He denied any other problems. He was by now fully orientated, had no cognitive defect and displayed no evidence of delusions or hallucinations (which he denied ever having). His conversation was laced with expletives which were introduced explosively into the interview without warning and following which he would resume as if uninterrupted. He tended to wink and nudge the doctor during the interview.

Subsequent thyroid function tests were normal.

What is the diagnosis?

2.6

A 69-year-old retired bank manager presented complaining of tripping up while walking. This seemed to be due to weakness of his left leg. However, this was an intermittent problem with episodes lasting for up to 2 days over a period of 2 months and with no apparent factor precipitating each exacerbation. Talking to his wife, it appeared that he had been intermittently mildly confused for several months, on some days uncharacteristically forgetting his grandchildren's names, while on others he would be entirely normal. There was no history of trauma. He was otherwise healthy apart from symptoms of prostatic hypertrophy.

On examination, he had upper motor neurone signs of a left hemiparesis, affecting his left leg more than the arm. He was fully orientated and there was no evidence of cognitive impairment.

One week later, the symptoms and signs had completely resolved.

(a) What is the diagnosis?
(b) Give one differential diagnosis.

Case Histories Paper 3

3.1

A 40-year-old advertising executive was alarmed to be told by friends that her eyes were turning yellow. She had been diagnosed as having rheumatoid arthritis 2 years previously and this had been symptomatically controlled with paracetamol. Apart from pruritus which had been diagnosed as skin sensitivity to soap, she had been well. She gave no history of foreign travel, visits to dockyards, tattooing, recent sexual contact, or blood transfusions.

On examination, she was icteric, afebrile, with scratch marks all over her thighs and back. The liver was enlarged 3 cm below the costal margin. The remainder of the examination, including urinalysis, was normal.

The results of investigations performed were as follows:

Hb	13.4 g/dl
Wbc	6.7×10^9/l (59% neutrophils, 36% lymphocytes)
Platelets	182×10^9/l
ESR	20 mm in first hour
Plasma sodium	136 mmol/l
Plasma potassium	4.5 mmol/l
Plasma calcium	2.45 mmol/l
Plasma phosphate	0.84 mmol/l
Plasma urea	5.4 mmol/l
Plasma glucose	6.5 mmol/l
Serum albumin	40 g/l
Serum total protein	95 g/l
Plasma aspartate aminotransferase	134 IU/l *(normal range 4–20)*
Plasma alanine aminotransferase	108 IU/l *(normal range 2–17)*
Plasma alkaline phosphatase	780 IU/l
Plasma bilirubin	96 μmol/l
Plasma thyroxine	120 nmol/l *(normal range 70–140)*
Chest X-ray	normal
ECG	normal
Serum paracetamol	not detected
Hepatitis A and B screen	negative
EBV and CMV serology	negative

(a) What is the most likely diagnosis?
(b) What three investigations would you perform?

3.2

A previously healthy 58-year-old security guard working at a building site was admitted having collapsed at home. Five days previously he had become ill with malaise, anorexia, nausea, a dry cough and dysuria. He was prescribed trimethoprim by his doctor. Two days before admission he developed diarrhoea and headache. He smoked 30 cigarettes a day. There was no history of recent travel or contact with someone with similar symptoms. The family owned a pet dog and a parrot.

On examination he was unkempt, febrile (38.4°C), mildly dehydrated, dyspnoeic and cyanosed with a blood pressure of 100/60 mmHg. He was disorientated and had mild neck stiffness but a negative Kernig's sign and there were no focal neurological signs or papilloedema. There was bronchial breathing in both mid-zones and inspiratory crackles at the right base. The urine contained a trace of blood and protein + +.

Intravenous amoxycillin, metronidazole and gentamicin were commenced by the admitting doctor. His condition worsened the next day.

The results of investigations performed were as follows:

Hb	13.1 g/dl
Wbc	$14 \times 10^9/l$
	(86% neutrophils, 10% lymphocytes)
ESR	56 mm in first hour
Plasma sodium	126 mmol/l
Plasma potassium	4.4 mmol/l
Plasma urea	9.6 mmol/l
Plasma glucose	5.4 mmol/l
Serum albumin	32 g/l
Plasma aspartate aminotransferase	100 IU/l *(normal range 4–20)*
Plasma bilirubin	14 μmol/l
Plasma alkaline phosphatase	130 IU/l *(normal range 30–100)*
Chest X-ray:	patchy shadowing both mid-zones reticular shadowing right base
pH	7.41
PaO_2	7.60 kPa
$PaCO_2$	4.90 kPa
Lumbar puncture	normal
Stool examination	cultures negative; no parasites seen
Blood cultures	no growth

(a) What is the most likely diagnosis?
(b) Name two investigations you would perform.
(c) What two treatments would you administer?

3.3

Two months prior to admission, a 66-year-old woman presented to her general practitioner with a 1-month history of malaise. In the preceding week she had experienced an ache in her nose and under the right eye. A clinical diagnosis of sinusitis was made and she was given a course of amoxycillin. This brought no significant relief.

In the 10 days before admission she had become increasingly tired and nauseated. On the day before admission she had become breathless and coughed up a small amount of blood.

She had not smoked for 20 years and drank no alcohol. She took no regular medication. She had two daughters, one of whom suffered from rheumatoid arthritis.

On examination she was afebrile, her pulse was 100/min and regular, her blood pressure 145/90 mmHg. Her jugular venous pressure was not raised and she had no dependent oedema. Heart sounds were normal with no added sounds or murmurs. There were bilateral coarse crackles in both lungs. The urine contained blood (+ + +) on urinalysis.

Results of investigations were as follows:

Plasma sodium	140 mmol/l
Plasma potassium	6.6 mmol/l
Plasma urea	45 mmol/l
Plasma creatinine	1134 μmol/l
Chest X-ray:	bilateral diffuse alveolar shadowing; normal heart size

(a) What is the diagnosis?
(b) What serological investigation would help confirm this?

3.4

A 22-year-old man presented with severe central abdominal colicky pain. He had vomited three times and was constipated. Two days earlier he had developed stiffness in his left shoulder and was finding it difficult to lift items.

On examination, he was distressed and had a pyrexia of 38.0°C. His pulse was 145/min and his blood pressure was 190/105. His abdomen was tender but there was no rigidity. He had weakness (grade 4) of both shoulders (the left was slightly weaker) particularly affecting abduction. Power was not obviously affected more distally. Bulk and tone were normal, but both triceps reflexes were absent. Pinprick sensation was lost around the left shoulder. The lower limbs were normal, as were his cranial nerves, save for the finding of papilloedema.

Results of investigations were as follows:

Plasma sodium	124 mmol/l
Plasma potassium	4.5 mmol/l
Plasma urea	5.5 mmol/l
Hb	13.5 g/dl
Wbc	8.8×10^9/l
Urinalysis	protein + +
	blood −
	glucose −

(a) What is the diagnosis?
(b) What are two possible explanations for his hyponatraemia?

3.5

A 65-year-old man presented as an emergency with a 3 hr history of moderate pain of sudden onset in the nape of the neck. He gave a history of chronic moderate low back pain for many years for which he had been seeing an osteopath. He had also been told that he had 'too many fats in his blood'. On admission his blood pressure was 150/94 mmHg. There were no abnormal physical signs.

His ECG was normal as were radiographs of his cervical, thoracic and lumbar spine and chest.

Two hours after admission, the pain in his neck became suddenly much worse. He became pale and his blood pressure fell to 120/60 mmHg. The blood pressure was the same in both arms. Physical examination was still normal as were the ECG and chest radiograph repeated at this time.

(a) What is the most likely diagnosis?
(b) What is the differential diagnosis? (Give one only.)

3.6

A 35-year-old man was admitted for investigation of intermittent blurring of his vision. During these episodes his pupils would dilate which caused him great anxiety. He also had problems with his balance, for which reason he walked with a stick. He had no other medical problems and was on no medication. On examination, there were no neurological signs. His gait was non-diagnostic and he did not really need the stick.

While in hospital he suffered one of his attacks of blurred vision, during which it was confirmed that both pupils were widely dilated and totally unresponsive to light or accommodation.

What is the diagnosis?

Case Histories Paper 4

4.1

A 30-year-old West Indian male bus driver presented with a 40 month history of tiredness and polyarthralgia. One year previously he had had arthritis affecting the knee and ankle associated with a rash over the right shin. This had responded well to treatment with non-steroidal anti-inflammatory drugs. During the past 2 months he had used over-the-counter eye drops for itchy eyes. During the past week his right wrist joint had become swollen and painful and he had noticed breathlessness on climbing stairs. He gave a history of polyuria and polydipsia for the past 2 months. His last trip overseas was 3 years ago. He drank socially at weekends and smoked 15 cigarettes a day. There was no family history of sickle cell disease.

On examination, he was afebrile. There was conjunctival injection but examination of the fundus was normal. There was a red lesion with a crusty rim on the margins of the right nostril and small papular lesions on the chest. The right wrist joint was swollen and tender. There was hepatomegaly (4 cm below the costal margin) and inspiratory crackles in the left mid zone of the chest. Urinalysis was normal.

The results of investigations performed were as follows:

Hb	11.8 g/dl
Wbc	7.6×10^9/l
	neutrophils 56%
	lymphocytes 40%
	eosinophils 4%
Platelets	182×10^9/l
ESR	38 mm in first hour
Plasma glucose	5.1 mmol/l
Joint fluid	Gram stain negative
Chest X-ray	left hilar node enlargement and shadowing in both mid zones
Sputum	negative for culture negative stain for acid–alcohol fast bacilli

(a) What is the diagnosis?
(b) List two possible causes for his polyuria.
(c) List five useful diagnostic investigations.

4.2

A 27-year-old male aeronautics engineer presented with a 2-week history of colicky abdominal pain, borborygmi, intermittent fever and diarrhoea of increasing frequency producing loose mucus-containing stool without blood. Over the past year he had noticed occasional loose stools and was feeling generally tired. He had lost 4 kg in weight recently and had developed low back pain. There was no history of travel abroad. He had received two courses of antibiotics during the past year for upper respiratory tract infections. He had a steady girlfriend.

On examination, he looked ill, thin, pale and was febrile (37.8°C). The abdomen was slightly distended, tender, and there was a diffuse mass in the right iliac fossa. The bowel sounds were increased in frequency. The remainder of the examination, including urinalysis, was normal.

The results of investigations performed were as follows:

Hb	10.8 g/dl
Wbc	11.6 × 10⁹/l
	neutrophils 69%
	lymphocytes 29%
	eosinophils 2%
Platelets	352 × 10⁹/l
ESR	56 mm in first hour
Plasma sodium	138 mmol/l
Plasma potassium	3.9 mmol/l
Plasma urea	4.9 mmol/l
Serum C-reactive protein	66 mg/l (normal range <5 mg/l)
Serum albumin	32 g/l
Plasma aspartate aminotransferase	38 IU/l (normal range 4–20)
Plasma alanine aminotransferase	90 IU/l (normal range 2–17)
Plasma bilirubin	7 μmol/l
Plasma alkaline phosphatase	82 IU/l
Plasma calcium	2.30 mmol/l
Plasma phosphate	0.80 mmol/l
Plasma thyroxine	104 nmol/l (normal range 70–140)
Faecal analysis:	*Clostridium difficile* toxin: not detected No ova, cysts of parasites seen

(a) What is the diagnosis?
(b) Name three differential diagnoses.
(c) List three investigations you would request.

4.3

A 74-year-old woman with a long history of rheumatoid arthritis was admitted with a 2-week history of increasing anorexia, nausea and vomiting. Three weeks previously she had developed an itchy, erythematous rash predominantly over her trunk. This had then faded over a period of 6 days. She had stopped passing urine.

Her rheumatoid arthritis had been treated in the past with gold, but for the past 5 years her only medication had been various non-steroidal inflammatory drugs. She did not drink alcohol, but had smoked 20 cigarettes/day until 5 years ago.

She was confined to a wheelchair by immobility resulting from her arthritis. She was unable to feed herself because of severe deformities of the small joints of the hand. She lived at home with a caring husband who had given up his job in order to care for her.

On examination, she was slightly confused, but otherwise had no abnormal neurological signs. She had numerous excoriations over her trunk and limbs. Her pulse was 88/min and regular, and her blood pressure was 185/105 mmHg. Her jugular venous pressure was elevated 4 cm and she had slight dependent oedema. The urine contained protein (+) and blood (++), and on microscopy there were 1–2 red blood cells per high power field (hpf), 16 white cells/hpf and 6 granular and white cell casts/hpf. It was sterile on culture. The rest of the physical examination was normal apart from evidence of inactive rheumatoid arthritis.

The results of investigations performed were as follows:

Hb	10.2 g/dl
Wbc	11.6×10^9/l
	(normal differential count)
Platelets	223×10^9/l
Plasma sodium	132 mmol/l
Plasma potassium	8.1 mmol/l
Plasma bicarbonate	12 mmol/l
Plasma urea	45 mmol/l
Plasma creatinine	873 μmol/l
Abdominal ultrasound:	no evidence of obstruction; renal size within normal limits

(a) What is the diagnosis?
(b) What are your first two management measures?

4.4

A 43-year-old Asian male, non-smoker and teetotaller, was admitted with a 2-day history of lethargy, sore throat, runny nose and headache. He developed vomiting and became confused a few hours before admission. Three days prior to admission he had returned to London with his family from a visit to Tunisia. His son was recovering from a bout of *Shigella* diarrhoea. He had no history of allergies. A splenectomy had been performed on him a year previously after a road accident. He was on no medication.

On examination he was disorientated, confused, febrile (39.7°C) and photophobic. The blood pressure was 98/56 mmHg and the pulse was 110 beats/min, regular but of low volume. There was a petechial rash on the left arm and right thigh. He had mild neck stiffness, a positive Kernig's sign but the optic discs were normal. Urinalysis was normal.

(a) What is the diagnosis?
(b) What investigation is required urgently?
(c) What treatment would you prescribe immediately?

4.5

A 54-year-old female has been treated with insulin for diabetes for the past 10 years. She has been referred for investigation of recently diagnosed hypertension. She is currently taking 40 units of insulin in the morning and 30 in the evening.

Examination shows her to be obese with a blood pressure of 180/100 mmHg, measured using a large cuff.

Results of investigations were as follows:

Plasma sodium	136 mmol/l
Plasma potassium	4.1 mmol/l
Plasma creatinine	130 μmol/l
Plasma glucose	11.0 mmol/l
Serum HDL	0.7 mmol/l
	(normal range >0.91 mmol/l)
Urinalysis	protein + +

(a) What do you suspect is the underlying diagnosis?
(b) What is the best treatment for this condition?
(c) What treatment would you prescribe for her hypertension?

4.6

A 77-year-old man with a long-standing bipolar affective disorder, managed on lithium, is found to be hypertensive by his general practitioner, who commences drug therapy. Three weeks later the patient is confused and off his food.

Results of investigations show the following:

Plasma sodium	136 mmol/l
Plasma potassium	3.3 mmol/l
Plasma creatinine	95 μmol/l
Serum lithium	2.3 mmol/l
	(therapeutic range: 0.3–1.3)

(a) What type of medication did the general practitioner prescribe?
(b) Why does he have toxic levels of serum lithium?

Case Histories Paper 5

5.1

A 68-year-old lady of low intelligence was admitted following an episode of haemoptysis. She had been unwell for some days with cough productive of green sputum occasionally flecked with blood. On direct questioning she admitted to episodes of diarrhoea for several months. She smoked heavily, although this could not be quantified accurately, and drank a glass of stout per night.

On examination she was thin and cachectic. Her temperature was 38.0°C. Her pulse was 88/min and her blood pressure 150/85 mmHg. She had cv (systolic) waves visible in her JVP and a rough pansystolic murmur, audible in the precordium. There were widespread coarse crepitations throughout the chest. She had mild hepatic enlargement (1 cm) but no other abnormalities in her abdomen. There were no neurological features.

Her chest radiograph showed cardiac enlargement and multiple rounded opacities in both lung fields. These opacities were of differing sizes and had borders that were poorly defined. Hepatic ultrasound showed numerous rounded regions which were relatively poor in echoes. Full blood count was as follows: Hb 9.6 g/dl, Wbc 15.3×10^9/l, platelets 431×10^9/l. Biochemistry was within normal limits.

(a) What is the diagnosis?
(b) What two investigations should be performed?

5.2

A 55-year-old man was referred by his general practitioner with an 18-month history of increasing tiredness, weight loss, dyspnoea and dry cough. There was no history of musculoskeletal or skin abnormalities. He was a lifelong non-smoker who had worked in a factory for the past 20 years. He was on no medication. He had been abroad 3 times in the past 10 years, to Italy, Spain and Greece.

On examination he was a fit man who was dyspnoeic on moderate exertion. He was not clubbed and had no lymphadenopathy. He had fine bilateral crepitations which did not change following coughing. His blood pressure was 165/95 mmHg. The rest of the examination was within normal limits. He was unable to produce sputum for examination. Urinalysis was normal.

His chest radiograph showed reticular shadowing affecting particularly the mid-zones, being more marked on the left. His lung function tests (expressed as percentages of predicted values) were as follows: FEV_1 77%, FVC 60%, TLC 62%, RV 70%, K_{CO} 50%. Autoimmune serology was negative. Full blood count (including differential count) and routine biochemistry screen (including calcium) were normal. Bronchoalveolar lavage showed an increased number of neutrophils. Kveim test was negative and serum angiotensin converting enzyme (SACE) was normal.

(a) What is the diagnosis?
(b) What are your first two management strategies?

5.3

A 20-year-old Caucasian woman was referred with persistent severe acne and hirsutism. She had never had regular periods and her menstrual bleeding, which occurred relatively infrequently, was often very heavy. She was on no medication and used barrier methods of contraception with her boyfriend. Her mother had similarly never had menstrual regularity and had also complained of hirsutism in her youth.

On examination, she was obese, had moderately severe acne, greasy skin, and excessive amounts of body hair in a male pattern distribution. The distribution of her obesity was uniform. Her visual fields were normal. There were no other abnormalities on examination, including on urinalysis.

Results of investigations were as follows:

Plasma luteinizing hormone	20 U/l
	(normal range 3–8 U/l)
Plasma follicle stimulating hormone	6 U/l
	(normal range 2–8 U/l)
Plasma prolactin	423 U/l
	(normal range <600 U/l)
Plasma thyroxine	98 nmol/l
	(normal range 70–140)
Plasma testosterone	11 nmol/l
	(normal range 1–3 U/l)
Dehydroepiandrosterone sulphate (DHAS)	6 μmol/l
	(normal range 3–7 μmol/l)
Urinary 17-oxosteroids	39 μmol/l
	(normal range 14–59 μmol/l)

(a) What is the diagnosis?
(b) How would you confirm this?

5.4

A 49-year-old woman presented to her GP with a 2-day history of severe epigastric pain and vomiting. She had been drinking with friends to celebrate her birthday. The pain responded to a proprietary antacid. She then visited her GP again with recurrent heartburn and epigastric pain. When seen in the gastroenterology outpatient clinic she gave a 3-week history of weight loss and diarrhoea. Her maternal aunt had a history of peptic ulcer.

There were no abnormalities on physical examination.

An out-patient endoscopy showed two deep duodenal ulcers, one extending beyond the first part of the duodenum, but no *Helicobacter* was isolated. Sigmoidoscopic findings were normal.

She was prescribed cimetidine and at her next clinic appointment 8 weeks later she complained of persisting diarrhoea and epigastric pain.

(a) What two further diagnostic tests would you perform?
(b) What is the diagnosis?

5.5

A 26-year-old woman was admitted for an elective laparoscopic investigation of infertility. Unfortunately, the common iliac artery was torn during the procedure and an urgent laparotomy was required to staunch the haemorrhage. This proved difficult and she required two further urgent laparotomies in the next 24 h. She was now intubated and was being managed on the Intensive Care Unit. She became oliguric. This failed to respond to conservative measures and she was commenced on continuous veno-venous haemofiltration through an indwelling double lumen femoral cannula. She was also being given total parenteral nutrition via an internal jugular cannula.

In the first 10 days of her illness she had a mild continuous pyrexia of between 37.5°C and 38.0°C despite being given ampicillin, flucloxacillin and metronidazole. Her white cell count ran between 13 and 15×10^9/l and her platelet count was between 60 and 80×19^9/l. On the eleventh day, her temperature rose to 38.5°C, her white cell count rose to 20×10^9/l and her platelet count fell to 40×10^9/l. Her antibiotics were changed to ceftazidime and metronidazole.

Seventy-two hours later she is no better. There are no positive microbiological results from any stage in her illness.

(a) What would be your first two lines of management?
(b) If they failed, what would be your second line?

5.6

A 33-year-old man presented with a 3-year history of increasing deafness and tinnitus in his left ear. He thought that it dated from an occasion when his infant daughter had screamed very loudly into his left ear. He was otherwise very well and was on no medication. He smoked 20 cigarettes a day.

On examination he was well. His auditory acuity was grossly impaired on the left but the external ear and tympanic membrane look normal. On Rinne's test air conduction was greater than bone conduction. There was no nystagmus and balance was normal. His left corneal reflex was absent.

(a) What is the most likely diagnosis?
(b) Name two differential diagnoses.

Case Histories Paper 6

6.1

A 29-year-old Asian newsagent was referred with a 4-week history of recurrent headaches, backache, fever and lethargy. He had developed tingling and weakness in the right foot and leg. On the morning of admission he experienced difficulty in passing urine and retrospectively admitted to two episodes of blurring of vision over the preceding few months. He had received treatment for a slipped disc 2 years previously and had received steroid eye drops for itchiness 1 year previously. He drank 6 pints of beer a week and smoked 10 cigarettes a day. He had several social problems following the break-up of his marriage. He was taking paracetamol for headaches. His last trip abroad was 3 months previously to Kenya, where he kept very well.

On examination, he was fully conscious and had unimpaired higher mental function. Examination of his optic discs and cranial nerves was unremarkable. Apart from a full bladder, the remainder of the examination was unremarkable.

He was catheterized and admitted for investigations.

Later that day he developed paraesthesiae and weakness in both legs and feet. The findings were now of impaired hip and knee flexion (power grade 4/5), increased knee and ankle jerks, extensor plantar response in the right foot, and impairment of all modalities of sensation up to level T4.

The results of investigations were as follows:

Hb	13.3 g/dl
MCV	88 fl
MCHC	33 g/l
Wbc	12.7×10^9/l
	neutrophils 40%
	lymphocytes 58%
	eosinophils 2%
Platelets	156×10^9/l
ESR	62 mm in first hour
Serum albumin	40 g/l
Plasma aspartate aminotransferase	20 IU/l
	(normal range 4–20)
Plasma alanine aminotransferase	70 IU/l
	(normal range 2–17)
Plasma bilirubin	6 mmol/l
Plasma alkaline phosphatase	80 IU/l
Serum vitamin B_{12}	280 ng/l
	(normal range 200–800)
Sputum and urine:	negative for acid–alcohol fast bacilli
Urinalysis:	normal

(a) List two possible diagnoses.
(b) List four diagnostic investigations which you would perform to differentiate between them.

6.2

A previously healthy 52-year-old telephonist went to her GP because of intermittent epigastric pain radiating to the back, and weight loss over the past 5 months. Unresponsive to cimetidine and antispasmodics she returned to her GP with a 6-day history of itchiness. She had noticed over the preceding 3 weeks that her eyes and urine had turned yellow. She gave a history of polydipsia. There was no history of travel abroad, transfusions, or contact with jaundiced persons. Her last sexual contact was 4 years previously. Her weight had dropped from 78 to 69 kg. She did not drink alcohol.

On examination she was pale, jaundiced and afebrile. There was mild epigastric tenderness, hepatomegaly (3 cm below the costal margin), and her gall-bladder was palpable. The remainder of the examination, including urinalysis, was normal.

The results of investigations were as follows:

Hb	10.8 g/dl
MCV	80 fl
Wbc	9.7×10^9/l
ESR	77 mm in first hour
Plasma aspartate aminotransferase	48 IU/l *(normal range 4–20)*
Plasma bilirubin	172 μmol/l
Plasma alkaline phosphatase	474 IU/l *(normal range 30–100)*
Plasma glucose (random)	11 mmol/l
Urine analysis	bilirubin + + urobilinogen − glucose + +
Chest and plain abdominal X-rays	normal

(a) Which investigation is most likely to provide the diagnosis?
(b) Give two differential diagnoses.

6.3

A 40-year-old Argentinian waiter presented to his GP with shortness of breath. He failed to respond to two courses of antibiotics but did improve somewhat on thiazide diuretics. Six months later he was demonstrably worse and was referred to hospital for further evaluation.

He was now complaining of exertional dyspnoea and marked swelling of his ankles. Direct questioning revealed mild dysphagia and regurgitation as well as intermittent constipation. He was a moderate smoker but did not drink. He was on no medication other than the diuretic. He had previously had falciparum malaria. He had come to the UK at the age of 24 years and had returned to Argentina only twice since then. There was no family history of illness.

On examination he was thin but apyrexial. His pulse was 98/min at rest. His blood pressure was 100/50 mmHg. His JVP was raised to the angle of his jaw and the wave form was not visible. He had dependent oedema to the sacrum. His cardiac impulse was diffuse and displaced to the mid-axillary line. Heart sounds were normal. Respiratory and neurological examinations were normal. In the abdomen, he had non-pulsatile hepatomegaly and marked faecal loading. Urinalysis was normal.

His chest radiograph showed gross cardiomegaly. The lungs appeared normal. Echocardio-graphy showed globally hypokinetic left and right ventricles. There were no valvular abnormal-ities. ECG showed an intraventricular conduction defect with numerous ventricular ectopics. Twenty-four hour continuous ECG monitoring revealed four brief episodes of ventricular tachycardia. Barium swallow showed a dilated and poorly contracting oesophagus.

On the fourth day of hospital admission he had a minor pulmonary embolism for which he was anticoagulated.

(a) What is the diagnosis?
(b) Give one differential diagnosis.

6.4

A 25-year-old woman presents with bruises and occasional nose bleeds over a period of 2 months. In the middle of that 2-month period the bruising seemed to be less of a problem. She is otherwise well. Specifically, she had had no shortness of breath or tiredness and had had no recent infections. She was rather a heavy drinker, consuming 2–3 gin-and-tonics a day.

On examination, she looked well and was not clinically anaemic. She had petechiae on the ulnar surfaces of both forearms. She had neither lymphadenopathy nor splenomegaly.

The results of investigations were as follows:

Hb	13.4 g/dl
Wbc	$9.8 \times 10^9/l$
	(normal differential)
Platelets	$95 \times 10^9/l$
Blood film	normal
Prothrombin time	14 s
	(normal range 11–15 s)
Activated partial thromboplastin time	30 s
	(normal range 25–34 s)

(a) What is the most likely cause of this woman's bleeding disorder?
(b) Name two possible causes.

6.5

A previously fit, sensible 70-year-old man was prescribed ibuprofen by his general practitioner for osteoarthritis. He returned the following month complaining of breathlessness.

On examination, the only abnormalities found were changes of osteoarthritis. There were no physical signs in his respiratory system.

Respiratory function tests show his peak expiratory flow rate, FEV_1 and FVC to be within the predicted range.

Suggest three explanations for his breathlessness.

6.6

You are called urgently to see a diabetic patient who has become very unwell minutes after being given intravenous ampicillin for a chest infection. She started to wheeze and complain of chest tightness and abdominal pain. Her pulse is 125/min, her blood pressure 95/60 and she is cyanosed.

(a) What is the first medication you would prescribe? Name the drug, the route of administration and the amount to be given.
(b) Name three other management procedures you would initiate.

Case Histories Paper 7

7.1

A 21-year-old male history student developed jaundice. For the past 2 weeks he had felt unwell with anorexia, lethargy, muscle pains, and a sore throat. He had not improved after a course of erythromycin. There had been no change in colour of urine or stool. He had never been abroad. He did not smoke but drank one bottle of vodka at weekends. He had had several female sexual contacts within the past 6 months. His brother had Gilbert's disease. He did not keep any pets and had no allergies. He was on no medications and did not abuse narcotics.

On examination he was pyrexial (38.2°C), icteric, with several slightly tender enlarged cervical and axillary nodes. There was a 3 cm hepatomegaly and the splenic tip was palpable. He had a small tattoo on his left forearm. Urinalysis was normal.

The results of investigations performed were as follows:

Hb	12.6 g/dl
MCV	90 fl
MCHC	34 g/l
Wbc	11.8×10^9/l
	neutrophils 42%
	lymphocytes 56%
	eosinophils 2%
Platelets	56×10^9/l
Blood film	autoagglutination of red cells
ESR	42 mm in first hour
Serum albumin	38 g/l
Plasma aspartate aminotransferase	120 IU/l *(normal range 4–20)*
Plasma alanine aminotransferase	80 IU/l *(normal range 2–17)*
Plasma bilirubin	106 μmol/l
Plasma alkaline phosphatase	140 IU/l *(normal range 30–100)*
Chest X-ray	normal

(a) List three differential diagnoses.
(b) What four further tests would you perform?

7.2

A 67-year-old man who had suffered from rheumatoid arthritis for many years was referred for further investigation. He complained of 4 months' increasing tiredness and lethargy and was now experiencing nausea and abdominal discomfort.

His rheumatoid arthritis had initially been controlled with non-steroidal anti-inflammatory drugs and several years previously he had received a course of penicillamine. His medication now consisted of prednisolone 6 mg daily and indomethacin.

He had no other medical problems and was reasonably self-sufficient considering the deformities of his hands. He had continued to work as a civil servant until 2 years ago.

On examination there was no evidence of active arthritis. His cardiovascular and respiratory systems were normal. He had mild hepatomegaly and moderate splenomegaly. Urinalysis revealed proteinuria (+ +).

Results of investigations performed were as follows:

Hb	9.9 g/dl
Wbc	9.2×10^9/l
Platelets	101×10^9/l
Plasma sodium	144 mmol/l
Plasma potassium	5.1 mmol/l
Plasma urea	31.2 mmol/l
Plasma creatinine	499 μmol/l
Creatinine clearance	21 ml/min
Renal ultrasound:	kidney size at upper limit of normal; no evidence of obstruction

A renal biopsy was abandoned after several attempts to obtain tissue. Following the procedure he had a life-threatening haemorrhage.

(a) What is the diagnosis?
(b) How could you confirm this?

7.3

A 55-year-old greengrocer was referred with a history of several months of a hacking dry cough, particularly bad first thing in the morning. On direct questioning, it was clear that it had troubled him intermittently for at least 2 years. It was almost never productive. He also tended to be short of breath after walking only 100 yards on the flat, although this was rather variable.

He had never smoked. He had been prescribed salbutamol, ipratropium bromide, and beclomethasone inhalers variously for several years. Initially helpful, they had seemed to be much less useful over the past year or so. Two 1-week courses of oral prednisolone, starting at a dose of 30 mg, had brought no significant benefit.

On examination, he was dyspnoeic on mild exertion. His chest was hyperinflated. Otherwise there were occasional inspiratory and expiratory wheezes audible throughout the chest. His peak expiratory flow rate was 250 l/min. His JVP was not visible and the apex beat was not displaced. Cardiac auscultation was normal. The liver was palpable 2 cm below the right subcostal margin. By percussion, the upper border was in the seventh intercostal space. Urinalysis was normal.

Biochemistry and haematological studies were normal.

(a) What is the diagnosis?
(b) Which single pulmonary function test would you use to confirm this?
(c) What single therapeutic measure is most likely to improve his symptoms?

7.4

You are called to a cardiac arrest where you find that a 47-year-old man admitted earlier that week with a suspected myocardial infarct has collapsed in the corridor. You establish that the airway is patent but that he is not breathing spontaneously. You are unable to feel any pulsation in his carotid or femoral arteries. You instruct two colleagues to institute assisted cardio-pulmonary resuscitation while you await an anaesthetist and equipment.

(a) What ratio of rescue breathing to sternal massage do you request?

ECG establishes that the patient is in ventricular fibrillation.

(b) How many times and at what energy levels would you attempt DC cardioversion before administering adrenaline?

He fails to cardiovert following three cycles of adrenaline and a subsequent cardioversion.

(c) What are your next two management manoeuvres? (For drugs, give dosages and route of administration.)
(d) How long do you wait after pharmacological intervention before moving on if it has been unsuccessful?

7.5

A 30-year-old woman with schizophrenia was admitted 3 days after a routine out-patient appointment. Unusually, she has been increasingly withdrawn over the past 48 h and has been brought to casualty because her family is worried that she is now running a temperature. There is no further history available.
  On examination, she has a temperature of 39.3°C, with an impaired level of consciousness and generalized muscle rigidity. There are no other physical signs.

What is the likely diagnosis?

7.6

A 29-year-old man presented with a 3-week history of non-bloody diarrhoea. He had no other GI symptoms. He had a similar episode 5 years previously. It had resolved spontaneously. He had had three episodes of bronchitis in the past 6 years although he was a non-smoker. He had not recently been abroad. On examination, he looked well and was afebrile. It was possible to feel the tip of his spleen. There were no other physical signs.

Results of investigations were as follows:

Hb	10.4 g/dl
MCV	103 fl
MCHC	33 g/dl
Wbc	6.4×10^9/l
	neutrophils 5.3×10^9/l
	lymphocytes 0.7×10^9/l
	eosinophils 0.4×10^9/l
Platelets	87×10^9/l
Plasma sodium	141 mmol/l
Plasma potassium	4.9 mmol/l
Plasma urea	5.0 mmol/l
Serum albumin	28 mmol/l
Serum total protein	56 mmol/l
Plasma aspartate aminotransferase	30 IU/l *(normal range 4–20)*
Plasma alkaline phosphatase	115 IU/l *(normal range 30–100)*
Serum immunoglobulins: IgG	1.9 gl *(normal range 7.2–19.0 g/dl)*
IgA	0.1 g/l *(normal range 0.8–5.0 g/dl)*
IgM	0.15 g/l *(normal range 0.5–2.0 g/dl)*
Upper gastrointestinal endoscopy	gastritis
Gastric biopsy	chronic inflammatory gastritis
Jejunal biopsy	villous atrophy
	no *Giardia* seen or grown
Small bowel enema	normal
Sigmoidoscopy	mild focal colitis
Rectal biopsy	cryptitis with eosinophilic infiltrate

(a) What is the most likely explanation for his anaemia?
(b) What is the diagnosis?

Case Histories Paper 8

8.1

A previously healthy, 36-year-old lawyer was admitted with a 4-day history of fever, lethargy, anorexia and vomiting. Rigors, an erythematous rash over the legs, arms and chest, and pain in the right hypochondrium had developed the day before admission. He had returned 4 days previously from a holiday in Tanzania and Zambia. Before departure he had consulted the travel clinic, received all appropriate immunizations and had taken chloroquine and proguanil prophylaxis which he had continued upon his return. He had been bitten by several flying insects. His homosexual partner was apparently well. He did not smoke or drink alcohol.

He was fully conscious, febrile (39.2°C) and mildly jaundiced. He had a blood pressure of 130/90 mmHg and pulse of 102/min, regular. There was no neck stiffness and the Kernig's sign was absent. He had a macular, erythematous, blanching rash on the thighs, arms and anterior chest wall. There were two healing insect bite wounds on the right forearm but no eschar. He had oral herpes simplex, pharyngitis and injected conjunctiva. There was a 3 cm hepatomegaly, non-tender axillary lymphadenopathy and the tip of the spleen was palpable. Urinalysis was normal.

Results of investigations performed were as follow:

Hb	14.6 g/dl
Wbc	8.8×10^9/l
	neutrophils 46%
	lymphocytes 50%
	eosinophils 4%
Platelets	82×10^9/l
ESR	28 mm in first hour
Plasma sodium	130 mmol/l
Plasma potassium	4.6 mmol/l
Plasma urea	10.4 mmol/l
Plasma glucose	4.2 mmol/l
Serum albumin	38 g/l
Plasma aspartate aminotransferase	180 IU/l *(normal range 4–20)*
Plasma alanine aminotransferase	110 IU/l *(normal range 2–17)*
Plasma bilirubin	94 mmol/l
Plasma alkaline phosphatase	94 IU/l *(normal range 30–100)*
Chest X-ray	normal

(a) List three differential diagnoses.
(b) What five investigations would help make a diagnosis?

8.2

A 30-year-old male suffers from Crohn's disease and epilepsy. The inflammatory bowel disease proved very difficult to control over the years, requiring frequent courses of steroids. At initial presentation he was still having frequent episodes of loose, but relatively inoffensive, stool, but was otherwise generally well with no symptoms outside the gastrointestinal system.

He was taking phenytoin and prednisolone 10 mg per day. He has been a vegetarian since the onset of his bowel disease and has never smoked.

He was referred for evaluation of frequent episodes of cramp in his hand. At initial presentation, examination was normal apart from his being thin with ankle oedema.

Results of investigations performed were as follows:

Plasma calcium	1.95 mmol/l
Plasma phosphate	1.1 mmol/l
Plasma alkaline phosphatase	90 IU/l
	(normal range 30–100)
Hb	10.6 g/dl

(a) What single investigation is most likely to explain his cramps?

Some years later he was again referred again, this time because of a deterioration in his gait. His Crohn's disease was now quiescent with improved overall well-being and a weight gain of almost 10 kg and resolution of the oedema. However, he had severe proximal myopathy and had fallen several times, most recently down the stairs outside the clinic.

Results of investigations performed were as follows:

Plasma calcium	2.14 mmol/l
Plasma phosphate	1.35 mmol/l
Serum albumin	38 g/dl
Plasma alkaline phosphatase	1600 IU/l
	(normal range 30–100)
Hb	13.5 g/dl
Serum vitamin D level	36 pmol/l
	(normal range 38–101)

(b) What biochemical test would you request, and would the result be depressed, normal or elevated?
(c) Give three diagnoses.
(d) Name two further useful tests.

8.3

A 33-year-old male accounts executive with a 15-year history of insulin-dependent diabetes was admitted complaining of shortness of breath. He had never been properly followed for his diabetes because of poor compliance. He was known to have proliferative diabetic retinopathy which had been treated on two occasions with photocoagulation. His renal function had been slightly impaired when last seen 10 months before the current admission.

He had been reasonably well until 6 weeks previously when he had developed increasing weakness. Over the last week, he had become increasingly short of breath. He was a non-smoker and a 'social drinker'. His only medication was twice daily subcutaneous insulin. The only past history of note was a Ramstedt's procedure for pyloric stenosis as a neonate.

On admission, he had bilateral basal crepitations and had marked ankle oedema. His JVP was raised 4 cm. He was producing no urine.

His creatinine was 1133 μmol/l and he had small scarred echogenic kidneys on ultrasound. Chest X-ray was compatible with mild pulmonary oedema.

Four hours after admission a left subclavian double lumen catheter was inserted and he was commenced on haemodialysis. One hour later his shortness of breath deteriorated very markedly and he was now *in extremis.*

(a) What are the two most likely causes for his acute deterioration?
(b) How would you manage each of these?

8.4

A 35-year-old British chartered surveyor first presented to his GP in 1978 with a 3-week history of sweats, myalgia and lethargy. No diagnosis was made and the symptoms subsided. He presented again in 1982 with similar symptoms and with a single episode of minor haemoptysis. He was a non-smoker and took no medication. He had had no other previous illnesses.

Examination, including urinalysis, revealed no abnormalities.

His chest radiograph showed widespread nodular shadows. No acid-fast bacilli were seen in or grown from numerous sputum samples. A Mantoux test was negative at a dilution of 1:1000 and a Kveim test was negative. Serum angiotensin-converting enzyme activity was 58 (normal range <42).

He was given a complete course of antituberculous chemotherapy and simultaneously a reducing course of prednisolone. Neither produced any change in his radiographic abnormalities although he felt slightly better.

After 6 months he was readmitted for further investigations. At this time repeat Mantoux test and Kveim tests were still negative. His chest radiograph was unchanged. A bronchoscopic examination including transbronchial biopsy revealed no abnormality.

During this admission he had a generalized tonic-clonic seizure which was witnessed by the house physician.

(a) What two diagnostic investigations would you perform?
(b) What is the diagnosis?

8.5

An 18-year-old male was brought in to casualty by the Police, having been found collapsed in the street. They had phoned his employers (whose name was written in his diary) who confirmed that he had been totally well at work 4 h earlier. No other history was available.

He was cyanosed, had a temperature of 41.7°C and was generally floppy except around his mouth where he seemed to be chewing. His pulse was 165/min and his blood pressure 80/65. He had fixed dilated pupils. There was no neck stiffness or papilloedema and no focal neurological signs.

Results of investigations were as follows:

Plasma sodium	140 mmol/l
Plasma potassium	4.4 mmol/l
Plasma urea	5.5 mmol/l
Lumbar puncture	normal

What is the diagnosis?

8.6

A 6-year-old boy was referred with swelling of his left knee. He had played football in his school playground 48 h before and had not noticed any problems until the morning of referral. He had had no other problems. There was no family or personal history of significance.

On examination, an otherwise well-looking boy had a red swollen knee which was warm and moderately painful to move. He was not systemically unwell and had a pyrexia of 37.3°C.

Results of investigations were as follows:

Hb	11.8 g/dl
Wbc	6.9×10^9/l
Platelets	405×10^9/l
Bleeding time	normal
Prothrombin time	13 s
	(normal range 11–15 s)
Activated partial thromboplastin time	60 s
	(control 25–34 s)
Factor VIII level	123%

What is the diagnosis?

Answers to Case Histories Paper 1

1.1

Accepted answers

Acute hepatic failure (due to alcohol abuse) with the hepatorenal
syndrome (100%)

Acute hepatic failure (due to paracetamol overdose) with the hepatorenal
syndrome (25%)

Rejected answers

Hepatitis C
Alcohol abuse
Renal failure
Hepatic encephalopathy
Leptospirosis

Essence

An early middle-aged woman presents with
jaundice. A moderate smoker and a heavy
drinker, she has evidence of renal failure and
intrinsic hepatic damage.

Differential diagnosis

This question hinges on the differential diagnosis of her hepatitis. By far the strongest
clue favours an alcoholic aetiology. There are
no positive features to suggest an infective or
toxic cause. There are no positive features to
suggest paracetamol overdose, but it is always
important to consider this cause of acute hepatic
failure, so this answer would attract some marks.
There has been no febrile phase and her urinalysis
is normal, thereby ruling out leptospirosis. The
onset of jaundice is too soon after her arrival in
Ibiza to be linked to a viral hepatitis contracted
there. It is more likely that she increased her alcohol
intake on holiday. Given her lifestyle it would be
appropriate to mistrust a negative drug history.

Hepatorenal syndrome is essentially a prerenal form of renal failure which mimics hypotension as a result of the accumulation of
vasoactive substances. In order to maximize
renal perfusion, the central venous pressure
needs to be as high as possible. However,
given the tendency to lose fluid from the intravascular compartment, it cannot be too high.
For this reason these patients must be
managed with a central venous line. Since
hepatic failure is essentially a state of secondary hyperaldosteronism, the patient will be
retaining sodium – indeed, measurement of
urinary sodium, which will be very low in this
case, is clinically helpful. In addition, this is
the natural response to prerenal uraemia. Thus
the patient should not receive exogenous
sodium.

1.2

Accepted answers

(a) *Pneumocystis carinii* pneumonia with HIV infection/AIDS (100%)

   Pneumocystis carinii pneumonia (75%)

(b) Bronchoscopy, lavage, and transbronchial biopsy with silver (or immunofluorescent
   antibody) staining of specimens (100%)
   HIV testing (100%)
   Open lung biopsy with silver staining of specimens (as an alternative to broncho-
   scopy) (100%)
   (PCR analyses of specimens acceptable as an alternative to silver staining (100%)
   Induced sputum microscopy and culture (inferior alternative to bronchoscopy) (50%)

  (c) Trimethoprim-sulphamethoxazole (co-trimoxazole) – high dose and intravenous (100%)

Oxygen (100%)

Corticosteroids (parenteral) (50%)
Pentamidine (50%)
Dapsone with trimethoprim (50%)

Essence

A young alcohol and IV drug abuser, with recent syphilis and recent travel to Morocco presents with an acute febrile illness with features localizing to the chest, and jaundice.

Differential diagnosis

The clinical picture is of a respiratory tract infection in a high-risk individual with features characteristic of *Pneumocystis carinii* pneumonia (PCP): paucity of chest signs in relation to severity of illness, tachypnoea, cyanosis, hypoxia, and unresponsiveness to conventional antibiotic treatment for pneumonia. PCP is the most common infectious complication of HIV infection (for which this patient is also at risk) in Europe and the USA. There is no better explanation of the clinical features that would arise from either the history of syphilis or exotic travel. They should therefore be regarded as 'red herrings'. None of the other causes of pneumonia in the IV drug abuser fits the clinical picture so well.

Although the diagnosis is a clinical one, confirmation by demonstration of the organism is important. (*Pneumocystis carinii* is now classified as a fungus.) Sputum staining has a very low yield (although induced sputum is much better), but bronchial washings and biopsy allow silver or immunofluorescent antibody staining which has a much higher chance of identifying the organism. Diagnosis based on the polymerase chain reaction (PCR) appears to be more promising in terms of sensitivity.

This clinical picture is of sufficient severity to need parenteral treatment.

Choosing two (or any other defined number) of investigations
In real life you are almost certainly going to want to do many more investigations than the number allocated in the question. Be guided by two principles: (a) exclude anything dangerous and (b) display as much of your knowledge as you can – do not duplicate by offering two alternative tests for the same thing.

Pneumonia in the IV drug abuser
- Lobar pneumonias
  - classical   *Pneumococcus*
  - other   *Klebsiella*
  -                 *Staphylococcus*
  -                 *M. tuberculosis*
- Atypical pneumonia
  - *Mycoplasma*
  - *Legionella*
  - *Chlamydia*
  - *Coxiella*
- Fungal
  - *Candida*
  - *Asperigillus*
  - *Histoplasma*
  - *Cryptococcus*

1.3

Accepted answer

(a) Viral myocarditis (100%)

Cardiomyopathy (50%)

(b) Echocardiography

Rejected answers

Ischaemic heart disease

Essence

A young diabetic develops cardiac failure associated with non-specific ECG changes following a 'flu-like illness.

Differential diagnosis

The classical differential diagnosis of cardiac versus respiratory causes for dyspnoea is relatively easy in this case. The clinical features are suggestive of myocardial disease. This diagnosis hinges on the differential of subacute cardiac failure in such a patient. Her diabetes makes her susceptible to myocardial infarction, and although infarcts in diabetics are often painless (i.e. silent), she is young even for a diabetic to have major vessel disease of sufficient severity to cause an infarction. In addition, the ECG changes are non-specific, against ischaemic disease and in favour of myocarditis. Also in favour of myocarditis is the relationship to a 'flu-like illness. Having said that, the possibility of an acute presentation of cardiomyopathy remains, as this often presents during an acute viral illness. However, it is said that exertion during a 'flu-like illness (she was on a 'strenuous' walking holiday) makes the development of myocarditis more likely. The urea is raised as a consequence of cardiac faiure.

> Even although it is often possible to argue that the facts are compatible with another diagnosis, if one answer is so much better than any other, do not expect to gain any marks for anything else. The positive side of this is that you need not agonise over discarding a less likely answer merely because it has not been formally excluded.

1.4

Accepted answers

(a) Stevens–Johnson syndrome from one of several possible causes (100%)

Erythema multiforme (50%)

(b) Antecedent upper respiratory tract infection (100%)
Amoxycillin therapy (100%)
Son's chickenpox infection (100%)

Rejected answer

Behcet's syndrome

Essence

A young woman with an acute febrile illness associated with widespread mucocutaneous lesions.

Differential diagnosis

With all the classical features of the Stevens–Johnson syndrome – a systemic illness with mucocutaneous lesions in the mouth, conjunctiva and genitals – this is a clinical diagnosis. The combination of skin and mucosal lesions is relatively uncommon and none of the other causes usually present in this florid fashion. The combination of oral and conjunctival ulcers is also uncommon, suggesting Behçet's syndrome; however, there are no other features to support this diagnosis. The term Stevens–Johnson syndrome tends often to be used to denote a severe form of erythema multiforme. In fact it was originally described as being the syndrome of erythema multiforme, systemic illness and ulceration of at least two mucosal surfaces.

This case conforms to this definition, so Stevens–Johnson syndrome is a better answer than erythema multiforme.

> The general rule is to give as much detail in your answers as possible, e.g. always specify the side of a lesion. However, do not go too far. In this question, you cannot specify one precipitant. There is a clue to this in the second question – you are invited to provide three possible precipitating agents.

> Read all the questions in a case before attempting to answer any one.

> **Commonest causes of Stevens–Johnson syndrome**
> - Drug sensitivity
>   Sulphonamides
>   Penicillin
>   Salicylates
>   Barbiturates
> - Infections
>   Herpesviruses
>   *Mycoplasma*
>   *Streptococcus*

> **Causes of bullous lesions of the skin**
> Drug sensitivity, e.g. barbiturates
> Dermatitis herpetiformis
> Pemphigus vulgaris
> Pemphigoid
> Erythema multiforme
> Insect or snake bite
> Porphyria (porphyria cutanea tarda, acute variegate porphyria, cutaneous hepatic porphyria and congenital porphyria, but *not* acute intermittent porphyria)

1.5

Accepted answers

Random blood glucose using bedside re-
agent strips (anything slower is less
good) (100%)

Urea and electrolytes (you can get away
with this grouping, but 'biochemical
screen' to include calcium is too non-
specific; calcium would be in the next
line of investigations) (100%)

Full blood count (to detect a response to
infection) (100%)

Chest radiograph (100%)

Urine microscopy and culture (for maximal marks, you must mention microscopy) (100%)

12-lead ECG (100%)

Blood cultures (any other test aimed at
detecting infection is less good, in the
absence of any localizing sign, but this
will be slower than urine microscopy,
which is why it is less good in your
'first six') (50%)

CT scan of head (even if this is now to be
regarded as an easily available, early
examination, you would not proceed
with it without first performing normal
all of the above investigations and
finding them unhelpful) (50%)

Rejected answers

Skull radiograph (almost certainly
unhelpful, and although some still
expect it, the diagnostic yield is too low
for it to be one of your 'precious six')

Arterial blood gases (although patients,
especially the elderly, can by hypoxic
without being dyspnoeic, you would
wait until after the chest radiograph
before doing gases)

Investigations

As before, if you are asked merely for 'investigations', you must first consider those that will
help you rule out life-threatening conditions. Only then go on to list those that will allow you
to come to a diagnosis. If, however, the question asks for 'diagnostic investigations', you may
assume that life threatening conditions will have been excluded. One further tip on
technique: if you have a choice between six investigations that reveal six lines of thought in
your mind, or six that reveal only four or five, make sure you impress the examiner with the
comprehensiveness of your mental processes.

Essence

An elderly man presents confused with no
other clues.

Differential diagnosis

In this case the differential diagnosis is
extremely wide. The most likely six would be

infection, cerebrovascular accident, acute-on-chronic brain syndrome (i.e. dementia with a possibly trivial acute insult), clinically otherwise silent myocardial infarction, pulmonary embolism, and metabolic abnormality. The life-threatening conditions in which early further information would alter your management include metabolic abnormalities, particularly of glucose, sodium, or (less likely) potassium, head injury with occult fracture/haematoma, pulmonary embolism, and myocardial infarction.

1.6

Accepted answers

(a) What drug was used to treat the acne? (100%)

(b) First: CT scan of the head (100%)
     Second: lumbar puncture (100%)

(c) Diagnosis: benign intracranial hypertension (100%)
     Complication: optic atrophy or blindness (100%)
     Treatment: discontinue the precipitating drug (100%)

Essence

A young fat woman develops raised intracranial pressure after treatment for acne.

Discussions

This lady was prescribed isotretinoin for her acne. The clues lie in the fact that the GP offered contraceptive advice (isotretinoin is teratogenic and has a long half-life) and that the acne was severe but resolved on therapy: isotretinoin is the most effective drug for acne. One of the side effects of isotretinoin is benign intracranial hypertension (BIH).

BIH (otitic hydrocephalus or pseudotumour cerebri) is a syndrome of raised intracranial pressure in the absence of a space-occupying lesion. The cause is unknown. It may occur in the absence of any other pathology, usually in obese young women, or during pregnancy, and in a variety of endocrine disorders such as thyroid disease, adrenal insufficiency and hypercortisolism. A number of drugs appear to be capable of inducing the condition, including the oral contraceptive, vitamin A and the retinoids, tetracyclines, corticosteroids, and nalidixic acid. BIH presents with the symptoms and signs of raised intracranial pressure, which may be severe enough to cause progressive visual loss through compression of the optic nerve. Diagnosis requires exclusion of a tumour. The condition resolves rapidly with correction of any endocrine abnormality or removal of an offending drug. Otherwise treatment involves weight loss, repeated lumbar puncture, acetazolamide, frusemide and, paradoxically, corticosteroids. Lumbar-peritoneal shunting is a last resort.

Answers to Case Histories Paper 2

2.1

Accepted answers

(a) *Giardia* (100%)
Tropical sprue (100%)
Adult coeliac disease (100%)

Strongyloides (50%)
Capillaria (50%)
Clostridium difficile infection (50%)

(b) Duodenal aspirate and biopsy (100%)
Jejunal aspirate and biopsy (100%)

Rejected answers

Lymphoma
Schistosomiasis
Irritable bowel syndrome
Hookworm
Filariasis
Amoebiasis
Shigellosis

Barium meal and follow through
Abdominal X-ray
Abdominal ultrasound

Essence

A young man returned from the Far East, where he had dysentery, continues to have non-bloody diarrhoea and malabsorption.

Differential diagnosis

Persistent non-bloody diarrhoea following a course of co-trimoxazole is suggestive of a parasite infestation of the small bowel such as giardiasis, strongyloidosis or capillariasis.

Giardiasis is the most common and has no systemic effects, although that may also be true of other infestations. Since the stools are not bloody, both amoebiasis and shigellosis are very unlikely. Colitis due to *Clostridium difficile* is also possible since it may follow treatment with any antibiotic. It is not possible to differentiate an infestation from tropical sprue on the basis of the given information. Adult coeliac disease is difficult to distinguish from tropical sprue in the early stages.

Investigations

Duodenal aspirate and biopsy has supplanted jejunal investigation in many centres, although both are still acceptable answers. This investigation has the highest chance of detecting the histological appearances of sprue or coeliac disease and is more reliable than stool microscopy or the culture for the detection of parasites.

2.2

Accepted answers

(a) Reiter's syndrome

(b) Keratoderma blenorrhagica

(c) Blood cultures
Gram stain and culture of urethral smear
X-ray affected joints

Essence

A young man with fever, oligoarthritis of large joints, urethritis, conjunctivitis, and mouth ulcers.

Differential diagnosis

The history and clinical findings are suggestive of Reiter's syndrome but gonococcal septicaemia can be chronic and be easily misdiagnosed. Having said that, there is an 80% female preponderance in gonococcal arthritis, whereas more males suffer from Reiter's syndrome. The skin lesion on the foot (keratoderma blenorrhagica) is typical of Reiter's syndrome; in gonococcal arthritis, the skin lesions are usually adjacent to the affected joint which, incidentally, are usually in the upper limb. Reiter's syndrome in its varying forms appears frequently in all parts of the MRCP examination as do all the seronegative arthritides. The family history in this case is another 'red herring'.

Seronegative arthritides
Ankylosing spondylitis
Reactive arthritis
Psoriatic arthritis
Seronegative juvenile arthritides

Features of the seronegative arthritides
- Involvement of the sacroiliac joints
- Asymmetrical oligoarthritis
- Enthesopathy (inflammation at the site of tendinous insertions into bone), e.g. plantar fasciitis, Achilles tendinitis, costochondritis
- Extra-articular manifestations: uveitis, aortic regurgitation, upper zone pulmonary fibrosis, amyloidosis
- HLA-B27 association

Mucocutaneous lesions in gonorrhoea and Reiter's syndrome
Gonococcal
- Papules with haemorrhagic or pustular centre
- Petechiae (as in meningococcal septicaemia)

Reiter's syndrome
- Circinate balanitis (painless coalescing vesicles on glans penis)
- Painless mouth ulcers
- Keratoderma blenorrhagica (palms and soles): pigmented hyperkeratotic macules/papules/pustules

---

2.3

Accepted answers

Serum cyclosporin A levels (100%)
Microscopy and culture of urine (100%)
Ultrasound examination of renal tract (100%)
Renal transplant biopsy (100%)

Blood cultures (50%)

Essence

A renal transplant patient presents with a rise in creatinine shortly after transplantation.

Differential diagnosis

Investigations should be directed at revealing the cause of the graft failure, not excluding associated problems. Like all causes of renal failure, failure of a renal transplant may be classified as prerenal, renal and postrenal. It is reasonable to assume that the patient would have other prominent features of haemorrhage or hypotension; however, all anastomoses created at surgery (ureteric, arterial and venous) are subject to mechanical problems including dehiscence and stenosis. Renal artery pathology could cause prerenal uraemia.

The most likely intrinsic renal causes are cyclosporin A toxicity, rejection or infection. This early after transplantation, any rejection would be of the acute, potentially reversible type. After a few months acute rejection episodes do not occur but the kidney becomes subject to chronic irreversible rejection. The

other issue to consider is recurrence in the transplant of the original disease. Although diabetes may affect transplants, the only condition to recur early is focal and segmental glomerulosclerosis (FSGS). Postrenal causes of uraemia in transplants include ureteric obstruction and renal vein thrombosis.

Fever occurs in acute rejection and in infection. The lack of a fever excludes neither as the patient is immunosuppressed. However, it would be unusual for the patient to have no signs of systemic infection at this stage. For this reason blood cultures would attract fewer marks. The preferred initial investigations would be directed at the most likely diagnoses: acute rejection, cyclosporin A toxicity, infection and ureteric obstruction.

2.4

Accepted answers

(a) Pneumothorax (100%)

   Mitral valve prolapse (50%)

(b) Chest X-ray in expiration (100%)

   Chest X-ray (50%)

Essence

A young man with acute onset breathlessness and a systolic click.

Differential diagnosis

Answering this question depends on knowing that a systolic click can be heard following a pneumothorax. However, even without this piece of wisdom, you should be able to guess the answer. The patient is young and fit and has become breathless over the course of a day. There are very few causes of sudden dyspnoea in this age group, and although you might consider a pulmonary embolus, infection or asthma, you are given no additional

information to support these diagnoses, which more or less excludes infection and asthma. Pulmonary embolism remains possible, but is much less likely in this age group. Thus you are left to consider a condition which often affects young, healthy males with no prior warning and without other symptoms and signs. Put like that you should be able to arrive at pneumothorax. The only remaining problem is that you are not provided with any of the classical clinical features of pneumothorax. In fact, he is not very dyspnoeic and has a small pneumothorax. It would very possibly have been missed had it not been for the systolic click.

Given the relatively minor nature of the dyspnoea, it is possible to argue that this may be one of the mild symptoms associated with mitral valve prolapse – which also causes added systolic sounds.

Why pick pneumothorax rather than mitral valve prolapse? Why is it better to play down the lack of classical signs of pneumothorax rather than playing down the importance of the dyspnoea? This is one of the artefacts of the examination situation. The implications of sending the patient home with an undiagnosed pneumothorax are potentially more serious than failing to arrange an out-patient echo-cardiogram. In the real world this patient would have a chest X-ray whatever – but you only have one bite at the cherry in the exam.

> *If you cannot decide which of the possible answers is right, ask yourself which would be the most dangerous to get wrong.*

2.5

Accepted answer

Gilles de la Tourette syndrome with chronic self-inflicted traumatic damage to left con-junctiva (100%)

Gilles de la Tourette syndrome (90%)

Essence

A young man with self-inflicted eye damage due to obsessive behaviour, foul language and repeated gesturing, presents drunk.

Differential diagnosis

You either do or do not recognize the clinical description. This constellation of obsessive behaviour, often self-destructive, with foul language, tics and gestures are diagnostic of Gilles de la Tourette syndrome. The famous lexicographer Dr Samuel Johnson was said to be a sufferer, and indeed to have lost a job as a schoolteacher because his odd behaviour upset the pupils. The ocular lesion might just sound like severe unilateral cheimosis, as occasionally occurs in Graves' disease. However, nothing else is compatible with that diagnosis. Indeed it is **hypothyroidism** that is more associated with psychiatric symptoms.

2.6

Accepted answers

(a) Chronic right subdural haematoma (100%)

(b) Recurrent transient ischaemic attacks on a background of chronic cerebrovascular disease-associated damage (100%)

Parasagittal glioma (25%)
Supratentorial space occupying lesion (10%)

Essence

An elderly man develops intermittent confusion and weakness of his left leg, with documented fluctuations in signs.

Differential diagnosis

Confusion and weakness are compatible with cerebrovascular disease. Although it is common for signs of dementia to fluctuate, it is unusual for motor signs to come and go rapidly. Although the motor features could be due to recurrent TIAs, the association with confusion is less likely, unless one postulates pre-existing permanent damage on which the TIAs are superimposed.

Fluctuating signs are a feature of certain space-occupying lesions, of which chronic subdural haematoma is the most likely in this age group, and is a better answer than TIAs. The lack of a history of trauma does not detract from the likelihood of that diagnosis. Glioma would be less likely in this age group.

Answers to Case Histories Paper 3

3.1

Accepted answers

(a) Primary biliary cirrhosis

(b) Serum antimitochondrial antibody
Abdominal ultrasound
Liver biopsy

Essence

A 40-year-old woman with longstanding itching and rheumatoid arthritis treated with paracetamol develops obstructive jaundice.

Differential diagnosis

The history raises the differential diagnosis of pruritus and jaundice. Although pruritus may occur with any liver disease, it is more common with cholestasis. In addition, with the exception of the paracetamol, there is no clue as to an aetiology. The toxicology screen was negative and although this does not rule out a paracetamol overdose, that would be expected to cause a hepatitic picture of abnormalities in the liver function tests. In the absence of any other predisposing feature, the cholestatic picture (alkaline phosphatase raised out of proportion to the transaminases) in a middle-aged female leads to a diagnosis of primary biliary cirrhosis. This is a slowly progressive cholangiohepatitis with destruction of the small interlobular bile ducts. It is thought to have an autoimmune basis and it affects women more than men (90% of patients are females) with a peak incidence of onset at the age of 45 years. Nearly 50% of newly diagnosed patients are symptom-free. Apart from cholestasis and pruritus other clinical manifestations include hepatosplenomegaly, melanotic pigmentation, clubbing, xanthomata, xanthelesmata, arthralgia, fatigue, osteoporosis, osteomalacia, hirsutism and portal hypertension.

It is not possible to be certain of the diagnosis and the principal differential diagnoses are obstruction by gall stones, cholangiocarcinoma, carcinoma of the head of the pancreas, and sclerosing cholangitis, or indeed, any cause of obstruction. Gall stones obstruction is less likely without pain and the patient would be young for either malignancy. Sclerosing cholangitis usually occurs in association with ulcerative colitis. Hence none of these diagnoses is acceptable in this case.

Investigations and treatment

Plasma bilirubin and alkaline phosphatase are raised and liver biopsy confirms the diagnosis. Bile duct damage is shown by swelling and proliferation of epithelial cells and the ducts are surrounded by an infiltrate of lymphocytes, plasma and epithelioid cells. Granulomata, when seen, imply a good prognosis. There is a marked increase in copper-binding protein on biopsy. Antimitochondrial IgM antibodies are found in up to 94% patients and titres of >1:80 make the diagnosis more likely.

Treatment with several immunosuppressive agents has been tried but with varying success. Cholestyramine may relieve pruritus and vitamins D, A and K and calcium supplements may be required. End-stage PBC is one of the indications for liver transplantation.

3.2

<table>
<tr><td>Accepted answers</td><td>Rejected answers</td></tr>
</table>

Accepted answers

(a) Legionnaires' disease
   Legionella pneumonia

(b) *Legionella* serology
   Bronchoscopy with immunofluorescent microscopy and culture of washings

(c) Erythromycin
   Rifampicin (indicated in severe infections)
   Oxygen

Rejected answers

Mycoplasma pneumonia
Chlamydial pneumonia

Essence

A 58-year-old man presents with a severe systemic febrile illness associated with chest signs and chest X-ray changes, diarrhoea, haematuria and proteinuria, hyponatraemia and a raised plasma aspartate aminotransferase (AST).

Differential diagnosis

This patient has a prodromal illness with systemic symptoms, meningism and a pneumonia unresponsive to several antibiotics. Atypical pneumonias should be suspected when a systemic illness has a chest X-ray much worse than the symptoms (although this is not always true) and is not responsive to conventional antibiotics. This man's relative lymphopenia, abnormal liver function tests, hyponatraemia, with protein and blood in his urine, are all supportive of an atypical pneumonia.

Legionella pneumophila causes severe systemic symptoms often with nausea, vomiting and diarrhoea and even delirium or renal failure. Neutrophilia and lymphopenia may be present. The liver function tests are usually deranged, the plasma sodium is low and there is protein and blood in the urine. Treatment is with erythromycin and rifampicin is added in severe cases.

Mycoplasma pneumonia is the most common of the 'atypical pneumonias' and accounts for a considerable proportion of pneumonias presenting to hospital. The cough is often dry and there are several extrapulmonary features. Over half the patients have GIT symptoms, 25% have skin involvement (sometimes erythema multiforme), arthralgia, myalgia and 6% have CNS signs. About half of all patients have cold agglutinins and some have a haemolytic crisis. *Mycoplasma* usually causes unilateral consolidation although bilateral involvement may occur. Treatment is with erythromycin or tetracycline.

Chlamydia psittaci pneumonia (psittacosis if contracted from parrots, ornithosis if contracted from turkeys or pigeons). Again the story is that of a systemic illness with mild pneumonia or severe pneumonia. The chest X-ray shows bilateral patchy consolidation. Treatment is with tetracycline. Relapses are frequent and the bird source must be taken to a vet. (Pigeon fancier's lung is something entirely different. It is an extrinsic allergic alveolitis, and is not infective.)

Despite the association with a parrot, the clinical features in this case are better explained by Legionnaire's disease than by psittacosis or *Mycoplasma* infection.

3.3

Accepted answers

(a) Wegener's granulomatosis (100%)
   Microscopic polyarteritis (100%)
   Goodpasture's disease (or syndrome)
   (100%)

   Systemic lupus erythematosus (50%)

(b) Anti-neutrophil cytoplasmic antibody
   (100%)

   Anti-glomerula basement membrane
   antibody (50%)

   Anti-double stranded DNA antibody
   (25%)
   Anti-nuclear factor (10%)

Rejected answers

Churg–Strauss syndrome
Subacute bacterial endocarditis
Sarcoidosis
Miliary tuberculosis

Essence

A 66-year-old woman presents with sinus pain, breathlessness, haemoptysis, and other chest signs, haematuria and renal failure.

Differential diagnosis

Your initial approach to this question should centre on the renal failure, as this is the major 'hard fact' contained in the question. As well as renal failure, the patient has lung disease. She has a history of dyspnoea and a small haemoptysis, signs in the chest, and an abnormal chest X-ray. These signs are not very specific and should be interpreted in the light of the known renal disease. The differential diagnosis of interest here is that of the pulmonary-renal syndromes.

What is the nature of the lung pathology? Pulmonary oedema is a frequent finding in renal failure. However, the patient does not appear to be fluid overloaded as the jugular venous pressure is not raised, she has no dependent oedema, and the heart size is normal on chest X-ray. This makes pulmonary oedema unlikely to be the sole explanation of the chest problem. She is unlikely to have pneumonia as she is afebrile, although this remains a possibility; and although *Legionella* infection would be possible, it is ruled out by the length of the history. Finally, one comes to pulmonary haemorrhage. Everything is in keeping with this explanation of her chest problem, and although it is an uncommon diagnosis in the general population, pulmonary haemorrhage is not uncommon in patients with renal failure.

The differential diagnosis is now that of renal failure and pulmonary haemorrhage. In the absence of any other major feature, the three conditions that this association should alert you to are Goodpasture's disease, vasculitis and, less commonly, SLE. (There are a few other associations but these are much rarer.) Are there any further clues in the information provided? The history of nasal involvement suggests the clinical diagnosis of Wegener's granulomatosis, one of the vasculitides commonly associated with renal failure. Taken together with previous information, it is reasonable to use this 'softer data' to establish a diagnosis of Wegener's granulomatosis.

Bacterial endocarditis does cause rapidly progressive glomerulonephritis and cardiac failure. Right-sided endocarditis may cause embolic pulmonary lesions but they would not present a diffuse radiographic picture. It is very rare for sarcoidosis to present with renal failure, and then it is usually due to interstitial nephritis. Miliary tuberculosis would not fit with the chest X-ray appearance. Finally, Churg–Strauss syndrome does not fit as it is usually associated with asthma and it is much less commonly associated with renal involvement than other vasculitides.

Vasculitis

Systemic vasculitis can be difficult to understand, not least because it presents in a variety of ways to a variety of specialists. Although thought to be immunologically mediated, its underlying aetiology and pathogenesis are not understood and, as a result, a mind-boggling number of different classifications have arisen.

It is best to consider the vasculitides as an overlapping spectrum of conditions resulting in inflammation of different-sized blood vessels, sometimes associated with granuloma formation. This is summarized in the following table:

	Granulomas	
Vessel size	Present	Absent
Small	Wegener's granulomatosis	Microscopic polyarteritis
Medium	Churg–Strauss syndrome	Polyarteritis nodosa
Large	Giant cell arteritis	Kawasaki's disease
	Takayasu's disease	

The antineutrophil cytoplasmic antibody (ANCA) is an autoantibody present in various vasculitides. In general, it is most often found in small vessel vasculitis such as Wegener's granulomatosis, and less commonly found in vasculitides affecting larger vessels.

Antineutrophil cytoplasmic antibodies (ANCA)
Since 1985, ANCA has been useful in the diagnosis of the systemic vasculitides. It produces two different patterns of immunofluorescence on staining ethanol-fixed neutrophils:
(1) cytoplasmic staining (described as c-ANCA) is probably synonymous with the presence of an antibody to proteinase 3;
(2) perinuclear ANCA (p-ANCA) represents a variety of antibody specificities, including one to myeloperoxidase (MPO). c-ANCA is a highly sensitive marker of systemic Wegener's granulomatosis (WG) and is found at lower frequencies in diseases with incomplete forms and variants of WG. Anti-MPO antibodies are found in p-ANCA positive patients with idiopathic or vasculitis-associated necrotizing crescentic glomerulonephritis, particularly if they are also negative for c-ANCA, and in diseases not associated with granulomatous involvement of the respiratory tract. Anti-MPO is also found in anti-GBM disease and, possibly, also in SLE (at low titre). However, p-ANCA, but not anti-MPO, is present in some patients with other autoimmune diseases, such as ulcerative colitis, autoimmune liver disease, and rheumatoid arthritis.

	Sensitivity (%)	
Disease	c-ANCA/anti-proteinase 3	anti-myeloperoxidase
Wegener's granulomatosis (all)	80	20
Systemic Wegener's granulomatosis [a]	>90	
Limited Wegener's granulomatosis [b]	75	
Idiopathic crescentic glomerulonephritis	30	70
Microscopic polyarteritis	50	50
Classical polyarteritis nodosa	10	20
Churg–Strauss syndrome	10	70

[a] Respiratory tract granulomata, crescentic nephritis and systemic vasculitis.
[b] Without renal involvement.

Occurrence of p-ANCA in other conditions

Disease	Prevalence of p-ANCA (%)
Ulcerative colitis	60–70
Crohn's disease	10–20
Autoimmune chronic active hepatitis	60–70
Primary biliary cirrhosis	30–40
Primary sclerosing cholangitis	60–85
Rheumatoid arthritis	
with Felty's syndrome	90–100
with vasculitis	50–75
uncomplicated	20–40

Pulmonary-renal syndromes
- Systemic disease affecting lungs and kidneys
  Systemic vasculitis, e.g. Wegener's granulomatosis, microscopic polyarteritis
  Systemic lupus erythematosus
  Goodpasture's syndrome
  Cryoglobulinaemia
- Primary pulmonary disease with secondary kidney disease
  Bacterial pneumonia complicated by glomerulonephritis
  Legionnaire's disease
- Primary renal disease with secondary pulmonary disease
  Pulmonary embolism complicating renal vein thrombosis
  Pulmonary oedema
    Acute nephritic syndrome
    Acute renal failure
    Chronic renal failure

3.4

Accepted answers

(a) Acute intermittent porphyria

(b) Syndrome of inappropriate ADH secretion
    Excessive vomiting

Essence

A young man presents with severe abdominal pain, a predominantly motor peripheral neuropathy affecting the proximal upper limbs, tachycardia, hypertension, papilloedema, hyponatraemia and proteinuria.

Differential diagnosis

The coexistence of abdominal pain and peripheral neuropathy has a short differential. Diabetics may uncommonly develop a motor peripheral neuropathy and autonomic neuropathy may be associated with abdominal pain; the same may be said of lead poisoning. Arsenic poisoning may also be associated with neuropathy and GI symptoms. Alcohol may cause a peripheral neuropathy and is associated with pancreatitis. However, there are no other features to support these diagnoses and they would leave other features unexplained.

Guillain-Barré syndrome may be associated with peripheral motor neuropathy, hypertension and papilloedema, but the severity and dominance of the abdominal pain make it unlikely. Peripheral neuropathy may complicate GI malignancy, but the patient is very young and it requires a metastatic complication to explain the papilloedema (the peripheral neuropathy of malignancy is usually a non-metastatic complication). The best explanation of these clinical features is acute intermittent porphyria (AIP). AIP usually presents with abdominal crises and a peripheral neuropathy with hypertension and tachycardia. Papilloedema may also occur and hyponatraemia may be a feature of the syndrome of inappropriate ADH secretion. Similarly, about 10% develop proteinuria.

> Do not be tempted to try and pull together a disparate collection of complications of a common disease and its therapy when a single rare disease would do as a unifying diagnosis. It does not work in clinical practice and it certainly does not work in the Membership.

The diagnosis of the syndrome of inappropriate ADH secretion is made by finding a concentrated urine (sodium >20 mmol/l) in the presence of hyponatremia (sodium <125 mmol/l) or low plasma osmolality (<260 mmol/kg) and the absence of hypovolaemia.

Causes of the syndrome of inappropriate ADH secretion

Malignancy	CNS disorders	Metabolic
Small cell carcinoma of the lung	Meningoencephalitis	Porphyria
Pancreas	Abscess	
Prostate	Stroke	
Leukaemia	Head injury	
Lymphoma	Vasculitis	
Chest diseases	CNS sarcoid	
Tuberculosis	Drugs	
Pneumonia	Opiates	
Abscess	Chlorpropamide	
Aspergilloma	Cytotoxics	
Malignancy	Chlorpromazine	

3.5

Accepted answers

(a) Acute myocardial infarction
(b) Acute aortic dissection

(a) Acute aortic dissection
(b) Acute myocardial infarction

Essence

Sudden onset severe neck pain and relative hypotension with no physical or ECG signs in a late middle-aged man with a predisposition to atherosclerosis.

Differential diagnosis

Sudden onset severe pain above the diaphragm does not have a long differential. The most common causes are myocardial infarction, aortic dissection, subarachnoid haemorrhage, pleural disease (including following pulmonary embolism), oesophageal rupture, vertebral collapse (and other fractures), disc prolapse and the neuralgias and neuropathies. The pain of pneumothorax is rarely severe and is usually overshadowed by the dyspnoea. The absence of any other features confines the differential to myocardial infarction and aortic dissection – indeed, there are two predisposing factors for atherosclerosis. (Chronic low back pain is too common to be a valuable pointer to disc prolapse or vertebral collapse.) A normal ECG is entirely compatible with a diagnosis of infarction and normal chest X-ray and peripheral pulses are compatible with aortic dissection. Similarly, the site of the pain, although more typical of a dissection, does not exclude an infarction. Caught in a situation of being unable to differentiate between two or more diagnoses (partly implied by the question, unusually for this examination, by the use of the phrase 'most likely') it is reasonable to choose the more common condition – acute MI. The question allows you to reveal the other diagnosis in its next part. You would get good but not perfect marks for presenting them in the reverse order.

In the event, the patient underwent an urgent angiogram to exclude dissection and was found to have an acute occlusion of his inferior coronary artery. He did very well.

> Uncommon presentations of common conditions may be more common than common presentations of uncommon conditions.

3.6

Accepted answer

Clandestine self-medication with a mydriatic.

Essence

A middle-aged man presents with intermittent dilation of both pupils without other neurological signs and a bizarre gait.

Differential diagnosis

The flavour of this case, with one single objective feature, strongly suggests a non-organic aetiology. This single feature is accompanied by nothing else that would help place it in a recognizable clinical scenario. It is almost inconceivable that a central cause of bilateral mydriasis would have no other features. Given the associated feature of the bizarre gait, suggesting an unusual personality, the most likely diagnosis is that he was doing this to himself. In the event, we identified homatopine in his tears and he admitted to self-administration.

Answers to Case Histories Paper 4

4.1

Accepted answers

(a) Sarcoidosis (100%)

   Systemic lupus erythematosus (50%)

(b) Hypercalcaemia (100%)
   Central diabetes insipidus (100%)

   Diabetes insipidus (50%)

(c) Anti-nuclear antibody/factor (100%)
   Urea and electrolytes (100%)
   Serum calcium (100%)
   Biopsy of skin lesions (100%)

   Serum angiotensin converting enzyme
      levels (50%)
   Kveim test (50%)
   Bronchoscopy with transbronchial
      biopsy and bronchoalveolar lavage
      (50%)

   Liver biopsy (10%)

Rejected answers

Lymphoma
Bronchogenic neoplasm
Tuberculosis

Essence

A young man presents with a moderately long history of intermittent arthritis, skin lesions, dyspnoea and chest signs, itchy eyes, polyuria and polydipsia, hepatomegaly and anaemia.

Differential diagnosis

The clinical syndrome suggests a chronic systemic illness. Systemic lupus erythematosus could explain some of the features, but other features make it a less likely diagnosis: the patient is male, and the chest X-ray appearance would be rather unusual, as would be polyuria and polydipsia. It certainly should be addressed in the investigations. The most likely clinical diagnosis is sarcoidosis. The skin lesion is typical of lupus pernio and this picture of extrathoracic sarcoidosis is common in West Indians. Tuberculosis is not excluded by the negative stain for AAFB, but this clinical picture with tuberculosis would be unusual. Furthermore, one would predict that a patient with disseminated tuberculosis would be much less well and would have more florid abnormalities on his chest X-ray. Malignant disease such as lymphoma and lung carcinoma with secondaries ought to be considered, but again this constellation of extrathoracic features would be very unusual. Although the syndrome of inappropriate ADH secretion associated with lung carcinoma could explain the polyuria, this neoplasm is very rare in a man of this age.

Sarcoidosis is commonly associated with hypercalcuria and less frequently with hypercalcaemia. This can be sufficiently severe to cause nephrocalcinosis and polyuria. Hypercalcaemia alone can cause polyuria. Alternatively, involvement of the CNS with sarcoidosis may cause central diabetes insipidus.

4.2

Accepted answers

(a) Crohn's disease (100%)

(b) Ileocaecal tuberculosis (100%)
    Small bowel lymphoma (100%)
    Yersinia enterocolitis (100%)
    Actinomycosis (100%)

(c) Abdominal ultrasound (100%)
    Small bowel enema and follow through
        (100%)
    Colonoscopy and biopsy (100%)

    Serum B$_{12}$ and folate (50%)
    Plain abdominal X-ray (50%)

    One of the following, depending on
    your chosen differential:

    Stool culture for mycobacteria (ileo-
        caecal tuberculosis)* (100%)
    Yersinia serology (*Yersinia* entero-
        colitis) (100%)
    Laparotomy with Gram staining of
        biopsy tissue (actinomycosis) (100%)
    Laparotomy and biopsy (small bowel
        lymphoma) (100%)

Rejected answers

Inflammatory bowel disease
Ulcerative colitis

Inflammatory bowel disease
Ulcerative colitis

Essence

A young man presents with fever, weight loss
and non-bloody diarrhoea. He has a diffuse,
tender mass in the right iliac fossa.

Differential diagnosis

Superficially, this patient presents with a
picture not unlike a subacute appendicitis with
an appendix mass. (Remember the surgical
diagnoses!) But appendicitis is usually associated with constipation. The combination of an
acute illness with diarrhoea, abdominal pain,
fever, weight loss, anaemia, a mass in the right
iliac fossa, and hypoalbuminaemia suggests
Crohn's disease. Even in patients with Crohn's

colitis, rectal bleeding occurs in only 50%; it is
even less common in patients with ileal disease.
Lymphomas and infections such as tuberculosis, actinomycosis, and *Yersinia* enterocolitis
can mimic Crohn's but it is rare for ulcerative
colitis to present with a mass in the iliac fossa.
His low back pain is too non-specific to help.

---

*In practice, you are likely to have drawn a blank
on all other investigations before having the result
of this culture (it takes 6 weeks). At this point you
are likely to be proceeding to an exploratory
laparotomy. However, when asked at this stage in
the history about investigations, it would be inappropriate to suggest a laparotomy (unless you
were looking for a malignancy) but entirely
reasonable to suggest that you should be preparing
to culture for tuberculosis at this early stage.

> Do not forget to include surgical conditions on your differential diagnosis. You would be expected to have thought of appendicitis in a patient presenting with the acute ileitis of Crohn's disease.

> Asked for a diagnosis and a differential diagnosis in separate questions implies you have to put them in order of likelihood. That is not the case if you are merely asked for two diagnoses.

Investigations

Your investigations should reflect your confidence in your 'sole' diagnosis and attempt to define the extent of the disease. But since the question expects a differential, you would be allowed to investigate one of your other possible diagnoses. It would be reasonable to flag your concern with malabsorption by requesting one of serum B_{12}, ferritin, or folate.

4.3

Accepted answers

(a) Acute interstitial nephritis secondary to non-steroidal anti-inflammatory drugs (100%)

Interstitial nephritis (75%)

(b) Administer an intravenous infusion of calcium gluconate (or chloride) (100%)

Administer an intravenous infusion of dextrose and insulin (100%)

Commence (or refer for) dialysis (50%)

Establish the central venous pressure line (25%)

Administer an intravenous infusion of salbutamol (25%)

Attempt to establish a diuresis with high dose frusemide (10%)

Administer an intravenous infusion of bicarbonate (10%)

Rejected answers

Pyelonephritis

Attempt to reduce the potassium
Administer an ion exchange resin (such as calcium resonium)
Administer a fluid challenge
Administer renal doses of dopamine

Essence

A 64-year-old lady with rheumatoid arthritis develops acute GI upset and a rash and presents with hypertension, evidence of renal inflammation without infection, renal failure and hyperkalaemia.

Differential diagnosis

Your approach to this question should centre on the differential diagnosis of renal disease in a patient with rheumatoid arthritis.

Dealing first with the non-drug related disorders, renal amyloid is the most common.

Patients present with the nephrotic syndrome and progressive renal failure. A sudden decline in renal function might suggest renal vein thrombosis, as thromboses are a common complication of the nephrotic state. As there are no other features of systemic amyloidosis, this is unlikely. By contrast, glomerulo-nephritis and renal vasculitis are rarely a clinical problem in rheumatoid arthritis.

Drugs are a more common cause of renal problems in rheumatoid arthritis. Gold and penicillamine may cause proteinuria which usually resolves once the drug is discontinued. The renal lesion in these cases is usually membranous glomerulonephritis. Non-steroidal inflammatory drugs can cause renal impair-ment by a variety of means, including reduction of glomerular filtration rate (GFR). This may be worse in patients with reno-vascular disease. Alternatively, interstitial nephritis may occur. Chronic analgesic abuse, particularly with combination analgesics, may cause 'analgesic nephropathy'.

In this question, an important clue lies in the data obtained by urinalysis – white cell casts in the absence of infection suggest an interstitial inflammatory infiltrate, i.e. inter-stitial nephritis, or a glomerulonephritis. The likeliest cause in this patient are the NSAIDs, of which we are told she has had several. The rash which preceded her illness is also typical of an acute allergic disease.

Management

The immediate management must be to correct her hyperkalaemia. Examination reveals she is already fluid overloaded. But the level of overload described is not so severe that it should be considered life-threatening. The hyperkalaemia is – hence it takes priority. Calcium ions protect the myocardium from the effects of hyperkalaemia. Intravenous dextrose and insulin and intravenous bicarbonate sequester potassium in the intracellular com-partment, thus protecting the heart tempor-arily. Both these techniques (and of course dialysis) will lower the potassium in a few hours. Calcium resonium will take up to a day and is therefore too slow for a life-threatening situation. Recent reports have shown that intravenous salbutamol is an effective hypo-kalaemic agent. Intravenous bicarbonate is an inferior answer because it contains a heavy sodium load which carries the risk of precipit-ating pulmonary oedema.

At least one of your management measures must address the hyperkalaemia, although it would be reasonable to nominate two lines of management to deal with it. Calcium ions only represent a holding measure, so a calcium infusion as the only response to the hyper-kalaemia is inadequate. However, it is reason-able to omit the calcium (some clinicians might do so), prescribe glucose and insulin and give one other line of management. Similarly, prescribing dialysis will deal with the hyper-kalaemia. However, the patient is probably not ill enough to demand urgent dialysis, which is why that represents an inferior answer. Some marks will be available for stating you would attempt to establish a diuresis. However, you would not get away with a fluid challenge in someone as fluid overloaded, and in the real world infusions of high-dose frusemide are rarely effective. This patient has been oliguric for too long for dopamine to be considered. Because of the level of fluid overload, it would be reasonable to require a central line to manage this patient.

> Be specific. If asked for a management measure, describe what you would do, do not state a general principle.

4.4

Accepted answers

(a) Meningococcal meningitis (100%)
    Meningococcal septicaemia (100%)
    Acute bacterial meningitis (100%)

    Pneumococcal meningitis (25%)
    Haemophilus meningitis (25%)

(b) Lumbar puncture and biochemical and microbiological examination of cerebrospinal
    fluid (100%)

    Computed tomography then lumbar puncture with biochemical and microbiological
    examination of cerebrospinal fluid (100%)

(c) Intravenous benzylpenicillin and chloramphenicol (100%)

    Benzylpenicillin and chloramphenicol (75%)

Essence

A middle-aged man presents ill with upper respiratory tract symptoms, confusion, shock, meningism and a petechial rash on his return from North Africa. He had had a splenectomy and his son had just had *Shigella* infection.

Differential diagnosis

The clinical features of this patient are that of an acute bacterial meningitis. This patient does not have a spleen and, as such, is predisposed to OPSI (overwhelming post-splenectomy infection) with a number of organisms such as *Pneumococcus*, *Meningococcus*, *Haemophilus*, *Capnocytophaga canimorsus* (DF-2), falciparum malaria and *Babesia* amongst others. The first three of these are recognized causes of meningitis. The early clinical features of acute bacterial meningitis may be very non-specific and, indeed, may be associated with diarrhoea such as to suggest a diagnosis of gastroenteritis. The characteristic skin manifestations of acute meningococcaemia, petechiae and purpura (often appearing first in the conjunctivae and later leading on to skin necrosis and ulceration)

are occasionally seen with both *Haemophilus* and pneumococcal meningitis. However, they are so much more common with *Meningococcus* that the presence of the rash in this case makes it the first choice diagnosis.

The treatment of choice in meningococcal and pneumococcal meningitis is intravenous penicillin. However, chloramphenicol is preferable for *Haemophilus* infection. If your answer is meningococcal meningitis or septicaemia or pneumococcal meningitis, then you must answer the treatment question with penicillin. If you choose *Haemophilus* meningitis, you will not get many marks on the diagnosis section, but these will be even fewer if you do not choose chloramphenicol for the treatment. If, quite reasonably, you plumped for the non-specific 'acute bacterial meningitis', you must give your treatment answer as penicillin and chloramphenicol.

> If you pick out cardinal features of a systemic illness such as fever, photophobia, meningism and shock, do not be side-tracked by irrelevant information, however 'juicy', such as a trip to Africa.

4.5

Accepted answers

(a) Non-insulin-dependent diabetes with insulin resistance Syndrome X

(b) Weight loss

(c) Angiotensin-converting enzyme inhibitor

Essence

An obese diabetic on insulin develops hypertension. She has a mildly raised creatinine and proteinuria.

Differential diagnosis

You may be unlucky and get a 'viva' type question, where some knowledge of recent publications is expected. There has been considerable interest recently in the 'syndrome' of insulin-resistance, hyperinsulinaemia, and associated hypertension, coronary artery disease and obesity. In Syndrome X it is proposed that insulin acts as a growth factor for vascular endothelium, promoting atherosclerosis, and may cause hypertension through a renal sodium sparing effect. There is a characteristic fall in HDL. Without this knowledge, this is an extremely difficult question, although you should appreciate that the onset of insulin-dependent diabetes is unusual at the age of 44.

An additional complication is the fact that the term 'Syndrome X' has also been used in cardiology to denote ischaemic heart disease in the presence of normal coronary arteries.

The other piece of knowledge which you are being asked to demonstrate is that careful blood pressure control slows the progress of diabetic nephropathy, particularly if ACE inhibitors are used.

> Read the editorials of the *Lancet* and *BMJ* for the 6 months prior to your examination. Broadly, that defines 'topical'.

4.6

Accepted answers

(a) A thiazide diuretic

(b) Thiazide diuretics inhibit renal conservation of sodium and lithium is retained in its place

Essence

An elderly man develops mild hypokalaemia and confusion after starting antihypertensive medication. His serum lithium levels are too high.

Discussion

The likely candidates for first-line antihypertensive medication would include thiazide diuretics, β-blockers, calcium antagonists, and ACE inhibitors. Thiazide diuretics cause confusion, particularly in the elderly, and may induce mild hyponatraemia and hypokalaemia. They inhibit the renal conservation of sodium and lithium may be retained in its place resulting in lithium toxicity. It therefore is compatible with all the features of this case.

Thiazide diuretics

Effects
- Hypokalaemia

Implications
Arrhythmias
Digoxin toxicity
Routine use of potassium supplements is **not** indicated

- Hypomagnesaemia
- Hyponatraemia   None – usually minor
- Hyperuricaemia
- Hyperlipidaemia
- Impaired glucose tolerance (by inhibiting insulin release)
- Impotence (mechanism unknown)

Uses
- First-line drug for uncomplicated hypertension
- Treatment of hypercalcuria (causes renal calcium resorption)

Note
- Ineffective in renal failure as their action depends on excretion by the renal tubule

---

Answers to Case Histories Paper 5

5.1

Accepted answers

(a) Right heart endocarditis with mycotic emboli (100%)

(b) 2D echocardiography (100%)
Multiple blood cultures (100%)

Blood cultures (75%)

Rejected answer

Carcinoid syndrome
Secondary carcinomatosis

Essence

A cachectic elderly lady presents with an acute febrile illness associated with haemoptysis and chronic diarrhoea, tricuspid regurgitation, opacities on chest X-ray and hepatic ultra-sound, anaemia and leucocytosis.

Differential diagnosis

Given the cachexia, this is clearly an acute on chronic problem. The only other chronic feature described is the diarrhoea. Most other abnormalities (except the hepatic lesions) point above the diaphragm. The heavy smoking could predispose her to malignancy, but there are no other clues as to the site of a primary; the multiple opacities in the lungs and liver could represent metastases, but the radiographic characteristics would be very atypical.

The acute lesion is likely to be infective and the opacities in the lung are likely to be the source of the haemoptysis and purulent sputum. This suggests either that underlying lesions have become superinfected or that they are pulmonary abscesses. The radiographic features are more in keeping with the latter. The tricuspid regurgitation could be secondary to an underlying pulmonary problem. How-

ever, right heart strain tends to result from a pathological process that affects the lung fields globally. Multiple isolated lesions are less likely to do so. In this case the cardiac lesion is likely to be primary. If we postulate an underlying right-sided endocarditis, then all the acute findings follow on from that. We are left without an explanation for the chronic problem. However, the existence of a potentially immunocompromising lesion causing cachexia would predispose to endocarditis. Although it is more common in drug abusers, it also occurs on the background of general debility. There is not enough information to hypothesize further about the chronic problem. The hepatic lesions are probably due to mycotic embolic originating in the lungs and which have traversed to the left side of the heart.

Another lesion that has been suggested for this case is carcinoid syndrome. However, diarrhoea is the only other feature supporting this. One would expect a patient with carcinoid of sufficiently advanced stage to affect the right heart to be more generally symptomatic than this patient. Yet another explanation offered is of a *Strep. bovis* endocarditis associated with colonic carcinoma and causing

---

The major difficulty with this case is untangling all the strands and establishing causes and effects. Isolate one finding (preferably the least common or the best defined, such as tricuspid regurgitation) and analyse it separately. How do the other features of the case relate to it? If this approach does not work for the first feature chosen, chose a second, then a third.

also hepatic and pulmonary abscesses. However, the signs of right-heart disease mean you would have to postulate an uncommon complication occurring in an uncommon site. With a primary diagnosis of right-heart endocarditis, everything else follows on.

5.2

Accepted answers

(a) Chronic extrinsic allergic alveolitis (100%)

   Lone thoracic sarcoidosis (25%)

(b) Search for and eliminate any precipitating antigen (100%)
   Corticosteroids (100%)

Essence

A middle-aged man presents with chronic cough, dyspnoea and weight loss, reticular shadowing on chest X-ray and restrictive pattern abnormality on lung function testing.

Differential diagnosis

As discussed before, the first question to be asked in a case of dyspnoea, is whether this is a primarily cardiac or a respiratory problem. One may lead to the other, so it is important to sort out as much of the primary problem as possible.

> Remember that there are occasional causes of dyspnoea that may be categorized as neither the classical cardiac or respiratory cause, such as severe anaemia or hyperventilation.

In this case, the absence of any cardiac signs and a plethora of abnormalities related to the lungs makes this a pulmonary problem.

> Always consider lung disease under a number of categories:
> - Bronchial
> - Interstitial
> - Vascular
> - Pleural
> - Chest wall
> - Neuromuscular

The chest X-ray and lung function test findings make this an interstitial disease and the relevant list to process in your mind is the differential diagnosis of interstitial pulmonary fibrosis.

> **Differential diagnosis of interstitial pulmonary fibrosis**
> - Pneumoconiosis
> - Berylliosis
> - Extrinsic allergic alveolitis
> - Drugs, e.g. nitrofurantoin, busulphan, bleomycin, amiodarone
> - Radiation
> - Uraemia
> - Chronic pulmonary venous hypertension
> - Sarcoidosis
> - Histiocytosis X
> - Autoimmune diseases
>   Rheumatoid arthritis
>   SLE
>   Progressive systemic sclerosis
>   MCTD (mixed connective tissue disease)
>   Sjögren's disease
>   Polymyositis/dermatomyositis
>   Chronic active hepatitis
>   Autoimmune thyroid disease
>   Ulcerative colitis
>   Pernicious anaemia
> - Cryptogenic

Since there are no clues from the history suggesting that the pulmonary fibrosis is part of a multisystem disorder, or secondary to another specific cause such as one of the above drugs, we are left with purely pulmonary causes. (While it is true that certain of the autoimmune diseases may present with pulmonary fibrosis before any other the extra-thoracic manifestations appear, these would be classified as cryptogenic fibrosing alveolitis at this stage.) This whittles down the differential diagnosis to extrinsic allergic alveolitis (EAA), sarcoidosis, histiocytosis X, and cryptogenic fibrosing alveolitis (CFA). CFA is typically associated with finger clubbing. Although possible, the absence of clubbing makes this unlikely. Patients with histiocytosis X usually have no abnormalities on examination but have a characteristic bronchoalveolar lavage with 'histiocytosis X' cells. EAA may present as either chronic or acute disease, and in a significant percentage of the chronic disease,

no precipitating cause is ever found. Chronic EAA is the most likely diagnosis, and although the negative Kveim test and normal SACE do not formally exclude it, lone thoracic sarcoidosis is less likely.

Management

The two management strategies available with chronic EAA are an exhaustive search for and elimination of the precipitating antigen, and steroid therapy. For lone thoracic sarcoidosis, the only option is steroid therapy. If that was your choice in the first part, you are now stuck for a second management strategy. This confirms that the examiner was looking for chronic EAA as the answer to the first part.

> If your answers to one section makes it difficult to answer subsequent questions, go back and review your first answer.

5.3

Accepted answers

(a) Polycystic ovary syndrome
    Stein–Leventhal syndrome

(b) Pelvic ultrasound scan

Essence

A young obese woman with irregular menses presented with acne and hirsutism of male type distribution. There was a family history of this problem. She had raised LH and testosterone.

Differential diagnosis

Hirsutism is a difficult problem to solve. If hirsutism is not associated with menstrual irregularities you are unlikely to find an underlying cause. This woman does have menstrual irregularity. However there are specific reasons

to exclude most of the differential diagnoses. Her corticosteroid production is normal (DHAS and 17-oxysteroids) which make adrenal causes unlikely. Similarly there are no other clinical features of pituitary disease, making acromegaly unlikely, and her thyroxine level is normal. She is on no medication and there are no features of systemic disase.

The cause is likely to be ovarian. A malignant disease is very rare and unlikely, whereas polycystic ovary syndrome (Stein–Leventhal syndrome) is common – it is the cause of 80% of all cases of oligomenorrhoea and 25% cases of amenorrhoea. It is classically associated with greasy skin and acne as well as obesity and a family history is common. Levels of LH and testosterone are raised. It can be confirmed using pelvic ultrasound scan.

Excess androgens cause the hirsuitism and masculinization and excess oestrogens inhibit FSH and stimulate LH, leading to failure of ovulation.

Causes of hirsutism
- Adrenal
  - Congenital adrenal hyperplasia
  - Cushing's syndrome
  - Adrenal carcinoma
- Ovarian
  - Polycystic ovary syndrome
  - Ovarian tumour
    - Arrhenoblastoma
    - Hilar cell tumour
    - Krukenberg tumour
    - Luteoma of pregnancy
- Pituitary
  - Acromegaly
- Thyroid
  - Juvenile hypothyroidism
- Drugs
  - Phenytoin
  - Diazoxide
  - Minoxidil
  - Corticosteroids
  - Anabolic steroids
  - Testosterone
  - Progesterones
  - Psoralens
- Porphyria
- Anorexia nervosa (lanugo hair)
- Menopause
- Idiopathic
- Constitutional
  - Familial
  - Racial (e.g. Indian)

5.4

Accepted answers

(a) Repeat upper GI endoscopy
    Fasting plasma gastrin levels

    Secretin suppression test

(b) Zollinger–Ellison syndrome
    Gastrinoma

Rejected answers

Abdominal ultrasound
Selective angiography of the pancreas
CT scan of the abdomen
Barium meal and follow through

Essence

A middle-aged female presents initially following alcohol abuse with duodenal ulceration and diarrhoea unresponsive to cimetidine.

Differential diagnosis

20–30% of patients who have duodenal ulceration fail to respond to 8 weeks of H_2-receptor antagonist therapy. The other major reason for

its failure is non-compliance. However, neither of these possibilities explains the diarrhoea. In addition, it is unusual for simple duodenal ulcers to extend beyond the first part of the duodenum. The clinical syndrome of non-responsive deep extensive ulceration with diarrhoea is characteristic of the Zollinger–Ellison (ZE) syndrome, in which there is either a gastrin-secreting pancreatic adenoma or simple islet cell hyperplasia. 50–60% of these adenomas are malignant, 10% are multiple and

30% of cases are associated with multiple endocrine adenomatosis (MEA) type 1.

Diagnosis and treatment

The first requirement is to confirm that the ulcers have not healed, so the first diagnostic test should be a repeat upper GI endoscopy. The diagnosis of ZE syndrome is confirmed by finding a raised fasting serum gastrin level with a raised basal gastric acid output of >15 mmol/h. Fasting gastrin levels should be checked only after the patient has been off H_2-blockers and omeprazole for at least a week.

Alternatively, intravenous secretin will raise the level of gastrin in the ZE syndrome but will cause gastrin levels to fall in normal individuals. Abdominal ultrasound, selective angiography or CT scanning may localize the tumour, but this is a second line step following confirmation of the diagnosis. Treatment with omeprazole or high doses of H_2-receptor antagonists to reduce the basal acid secretion may help to heal the ulcers but neither these drugs nor gastrectomy alters the course of the tumour. Excision of tumours after their localization by CT scans or angiography may be of some benefit.

5.5

Accepted answers

(a) Change all the intravascular cannulae and urinary catheter (if present) (100%)
Repeat cultures after discontinuing antimicrobial therapy (100%)

Repeat cultures (75%)
Extend anti-staphylococcal cover with fusidic acid (75%)
Commence antifungal therapy (75%)

(b) Attempt to visualize any collections, first ultrasonographically and then at laparotomy (100%)

Essence

Following surgery, a young woman has a severe recurrent intra-abdominal arterial bleed and develops renal failure. She has a fever and thrombocytopenia, and fails to respond to antibiotics.

Management

Pure management problems are not rare in the grey cases: they will usually be testing principles of management. This woman has had instrumentation to and bleeding in her abdomen and continues to have intravenous cannulae. The problem now is one of unexplained fever and thrombocytopenia. The differential of the fever lies between a resolving haematoma and a collection of pus. Even if she does have a resolving haematoma, it may very well be infected. Certainly she has been too ill for too long to work on that basis. You must assume that she has an infection. Infected lines may be impossible to sterilize so should be changed. If that fails it may be necessary to stop her antibiotics in order to repeat cultures when there is a higher chance of their growing an organism. It is reasonable to consider organisms that may not be responsive to the chemotherapy used – particularly fungi. Finally, attempts to localize collections of pus should start with ultrasound and move on to CT scanning. If all else fails she will need an exploratory laparatomy.

5.6

Accepted answers

(a) Acoustic neuroma

(b) Basilar artery aneurysm
    Meningioma

Rejected answers

Multiple sclerosis
Astrocytoma
Glioma
Nasopharyngeal carcinoma

Essence

A young man with a 3-year history of increasing sensorineural deafness and tinnitus has lost his ipsilateral corneal reflex.

Differential diagnosis

The coexistence of the lost corneal reflex with sensorineural deafness and tinnitus means either there is a single lesion in the cerebello-pontine angle or there are multiple lesions. No single central lesion will cause these two features alone and it is highly unlikely that two lesions in the brain stem would cause these features alone with loss of only the corneal reflex. Do not succumb to the temptation to discount the corneal reflex just because *you* may find it a difficult sign to be sure of.

> If you are told that the patient has a physical sign – he has that sign. The fact that you personally find the sign difficult to elicit is not a cause for doubting its validity.

The most common lesion in the cerebello-pontine angle is an acoustic neuroma. Although it usually arises from the vestibular division of the eighth nerve, deafness and tinnitus are the earliest clinical features. Similarly, the most vulnerable of the other cranial nerves in the region are those fibres of the fifth carrying corneal sensation. Later on, a more extensive area of hemianaesthesia, hemifacial spasm, attacks of vertigo, ataxia, and spastic paraparesis may occur. Indeed, limb signs usually come to overshadow relatively trivial cranial nerve features.

The differential diagnosis is with other lesions in the cerebello-pontine angle. Lesions arising within the pons which could produce these clinical features, such as multiple sclerosis, pontine glioma (usually in young boys) and astrocytoma, are likely to present with more complex neurological signs. Extrinsic lesions, such as meningioma, haemangioblastomas, cholesteatomas, basilar artery aneurysms, neuromas of other cranial nerves, medulloblastoma, nasopharyngeal carcinoma, metastatic carcinoma and lymphoma, are more likely to pick off isolated cranial nerves. However, most of these are likely to present first with other clinical features, and are made more or less likely by the age of the patient.

Answers to Case Histories Paper 6

6.1

Accepted answers

(a) Pott's disease of the spine
    Tuberculosis of the spine
    Epidural abscess
    Multiple sclerosis

(b) Four of the following:
    Plain radiograph of the spine
    MRI scan (intracranial and spinal cord)
    Lumbar puncture with culture and electrophoresis
    Myelogram
    Visual evoked potentials

Rejected answer

Spinal/vertebral abscess
Spinal cord tumour

Essence

A young man subacutely develops upper motor neurone and sensory signs to T4 and bladder problems after a 1-month history of backache and non-specific symptoms and 3 months after a trip to Kenya.

Differential diagnosis

There are some features of the history that may be misleading (e.g. slipped disc 2 years ago, paracetamol intake). However, the essential feature is that of a spinal cord lesion which, at this age, may have several causes.

Causes of weak legs with spasticity	
• Cord compression	*Mycoplasma*
Disc prolapse at L1–L2 or higher	Mumps
Tumours	Measles
Vertebral fractures	EBV
Epidural abscess	HIV
Spinal TB	HTLV-1
Hodgkin's disease	Neurotoxins
Myeloma	Carcinomatous meningitis
Paget's disease	B_{12} deficiency
Schistosomiasis	• Cord infarction
Neurocysticercosis	Vasculitis
Hydatid cyst	Polyarteritis
• Myelitis	Syphilis
Multiple sclerosis	Anterior spinal artery thrombosis
Infective	Trauma
Tuberculous meningitis	Compression
Syphilis	Dissection of aortic aneurysm

The Asian background, raised ESR, raised white count with a lymphocytosis support a diagnosis of Pott's disease of the spine. However, in view of the neurological symptoms and signs compatible with a transverse myelitis and a history of blurred vision, multiple sclerosis must be considered. An epidural abscess is another possibility, as these patients may be surprisingly well. The history is rather rapid to be suggestive of a tumour, and the fact that the patient is not systemically ill makes a pyogenic abscess less likely.

6.2

Accepted answers

(a) Endoscopic retrograde cholangiopancreatogram (ERCP)
    CT scan upper abdomen

(b) Carcinoma head of pancreas
    Cholangiocarcinoma
    Secondaries to porta hepatis

Essence

A middle-aged woman presents with chronic epigastric pain and weight loss and now with pruritus and cholestatic jaundice.

> Even if the question does not ask for a differential diagnosis initially (or at all), that is what you should be considering in every question.

Differential diagnosis

The combination of cholestatic jaundice, anaemia, high ESR, palpable gall-bladder, diabetes and bilirubin in the urine suggests an obstructive jaundice, most likely due to malignancy. The candidate sites are carcinoma of the head of pancreas, bile ducts or secondaries to the porta hepatis. 60% of pancreatic tumours involve the head of the pancreas, 25% the ampulla, and 15% the tail. Usually enough B cells survive to maintian normoglycaemia, but frank diabetes may occur. It is unlikely that this picture is due to gall stones since a fibrotic reaction is excited by the stones and thus the gall-bladder becomes impalpable.

The highest diagnostic yield will come from an endoscopic retrograde cholangiopancreatogram (ERCP). In practice, patients are likely to have an ultrasound examination first and if the lesion is thought to be hilar, a CT scan of the abdomen also. They will then proceed to ERCP even if the diagnosis has already been made as this allows a stent to be inserted. However, the ultrasound scan may not be diagnostic.

6.3

Accepted answers

(a) Chagas' disease

(b) Systemic sclerosis

Rejected answer

Dilated (congestive) cardiomyopathy

Essence

A South American presenting with chronic cardiac failure, abnormal oesophageal motility, constipation and pulmonary embolism.

Differential diagnosis

The most prominent feature of this condition is cardiac failure. Most of the clinical features, including the hepatomegaly, are part of the syndrome of cardiac failure. The dysphagia could also have been part of that syndrome, but for the marked abnormality of the barium swallow which demonstrates that it is an independent phenomenon.

The echocardiogram demonstrates that the cause of the cardiac failure is a global myopathy, thus all but excluding an ischaemic cause. The differential includes causes of cardiac myopathy with disordered oesophageal motility.

The most likely diagnosis is Chagas' disease or chronic infection with *Trypanosoma cruzi.* No other diagnosis takes advantages of all the information, and it the only explanation which makes his geographical origins significant. The fact that he has been away from Argentina is

of no relevance since Chagas' disease is the end point of a chronic infection, usually acquired in childhood.

(Pan) systemic sclerosis or scleroderma (a less appropriate term) would explain the combination of cardiac myopathy and oesophageal abnormality. However, it would be relatively rare to have such a severe systemic presentation in the absence of any cutaneous lesions. A primary cardiomyopathy is occasionally associated with skeletal muscle abnormalities, but clinical oesophageal disease is not a recognized feature. In this case the echocardiographic abnormalities are compatible only with a dilated (congestive) cardiomyopathy which does not explain the oesophageal abnormality.

6.4

Accepted answers

(a) Acquired platelet defect
   Fluctuating thrombocytopenia

(b) Aspirin/dipyridamole/sulphapyrazone
   therapy
   Hypergammaglobulinaemia
   Uraemia

Rejected answer

Defect of clotting system

Essence

A young woman with chronic bruising and nose bleeds and who is a heavy drinker has mild thrombocytopenia and no disorders of clotting.

Differential diagnosis

Pathological bleeding is due to abnormal vessels, platelets or clotting factors. There is nothing to suggest a problem with her vasculature and tests show her clotting system is normal. She has thrombocytopenia, but it is too mild at the time of testing to cause spontaneous bleeding. However, that does not

exclude fluctuating thrombocytopenia, and indeed the type of bleeding is characteristic of that due to platelet deficiency. The platelet defect may be absolute, due to reduced numbers, or functional, due, for example, to aspirin or sulphinpyrazone therapy, hypergammaglobulinaemia, uraemia, or liver disease. The platelets produced in myeloproliferative disease may be functionally abnormal.

The most important diagnosis to exclude must be a proliferative disorder, but the absence of any other abnormality clinically or in the blood picture makes a leukaemia or lymphoma very unlikely. Thus an isolated platelet deficiency is probably the cause and given the history is very unlikely to be a congenital problem. Beyond that there are few clues, which makes this a difficult question. A normal prothrombin time makes significant liver disease less likely.

6.5

Accepted answers

Asthma, precipitated by the anti-inflammatory medication
Fluid retention, again induced by the drug
Anaemia due to gastrointestinal haemorrhage induced by the medication

Essence

An elderly man becomes breathless after receiving a non-steroidal anti-inflammatory drug (NSAID).

Discussion

You are given so little information that this question can be reduced to the side-effects of ibuprofen. NSAIDs, not only aspirin, can precipitate bronchospasm by their inhibition of the metabolism of arachidonic acid by cyclo-oxygenase. Production of bronchodilator prostocyclins is inhibited and bronchospasm ensues. Asthma is a reversible and intermittent condition, so that respiratory function tests may be normal. NSAIDs also cause fluid retention or may cause GI haemorrhage.

6.6

Accepted answers

(a) Adrenaline 0.5–1.0 ml 1:1000 subcutaneously

(b) Oxygen by face mask
H_1 antagonist intravenously
Establish central venous access and administer fluids to maintain venous pressure

Essence

A patient develops anaphylactic shock and becomes cyanosed.

Management

This is one of the few cases in which you will be expected to know doses of drugs. The first drug to be given is adrenaline. It can be given intramuscularly or subcutaneously, but not intravenously. You should give 0.5–1.0 ml of a 1:1000 dilution. The dose is the least important part of this answer. The patient is cyanosed – she needs oxygen. Give her 35%. Do not forget to mention it – even although the nurse will probably have the mask on the patient long before you get there. The second agent to be given is an antihistamine – it does not really matter which one. Chlorpheniramine is particularly popular. Given that she is shocked, your final answer should be to set up central venous access and administer fluid.

Any other management measure is 'second line', e.g. aminophylline infusion or starting a course of hydrocortisone. Other measures, such as intubation and artificial ventilation or use of an inotrope, would only be justified after the above measures failed.

Answers to Case Histories Paper 7

7.1

Accepted answers

(a) Epstein–Barr virus (100%)
Cytomegalovirus (100%)
Toxoplasmosis (100%)
Hepatitis B (100%)
Hepatitis C (100%)
HIV seroconversion illness (100%)

(b) Paul–Bunnell test or Monospot™ (100%)
or EBV IgM antibodies (100%)
CMV serology (100%)
Toxoplasma dye test (100%)
Hepatitis serology (100%)
HBsAg (100%)
HIV test after counselling (100%)

HIV test (75%)

Direct Coombs' test (50%)
Blood culture (50%)
Liver biopsy (50%)
Lymph node biopsy (50%)

Essence

A young man, whose brother has Gilbert's syndrome, develops hepatocellular jaundice, hepatosplenomegaly and lymphadenopathy after a 'flu-like illness.

Differential diagnosis

The clinical picture of anaemia, thrombocytopenia, presence of a cold agglutinin, lymphocytosis, jaundice, hepatosplenomegaly, and lymphadenopathy may indicate any of the 'infectious mononucleoses' (EBV, CMV, HIV, toxoplasmosis or hepatitis B). The biochemistry excludes obstructive jaundice and the clinical picture is not that of Gilbert's disease – unconjugated hyperbilirubinaemia in the absence of any sign of liver disease or haemolysis – even though there is a strong familial tendency. He had never been abroad and thus brucellosis is unlikely. Lymphoma and leukaemia must be looked for if the initial infection screen proves to be negative. The presence of a tattoo and several sexual contacts represent risk factors for the hepatitis viruses.

7.2

Accepted answers

(a) Systemic amyloidosis secondary to rheumatoid arthritis (100%)
AA amyloidosis secondary to rheumatoid arthritis (100%)

Renal amyloid (75%)

Amyloidosis (75%)

(b) Deep rectal biopsy with Congo red staining

Essence

A 67-year-old with chronic rheumatoid arthritis, previously on penicillamine and now on steroids and indomethacin, has non-specific symptoms, hepatosplenomegaly, proteinuria and renal failure. He bled following a renal biopsy.

Differential diagnosis

There are three 'hard facts' in this case: renal failure, rheumatoid arthritis, and hepatosplenomegaly. This triad makes amyloid the only likely explanation. Do not be thrown by the drug history – drugs are not the only cause of problems.

For a discussion of renal disease in rheumatoid arthritis, see page 57.

Note also that amyloid infiltration can make tissues more prone to haemorrhage and may have predisposed to the haemorrhage post-renal biopsy.

Recently, the serum amyloid P (SAP) scan has been introduced. This is not yet widely available, and there is as yet insufficient experience to advocate its use as the sole diagnostic test. Hence it is reasonable still to require a tissue diagnosis. The diagnostic yield from lip or gingival biposy is lower than that from rectal biopsy.

7.3

Accepted answers

(a) Chronic asthma

(b) Transfer factor (DL_{CO})
FEV_1/FVC before and after brochodilators
Peak expiratory flow rate before and after brochodilators

(c) High dose prolonged course of oral corticosteroids

Rejected answer

Chronic obstructive airways disease (with reversibility)

Essence

Chronic early morning non-productive cough and exertional dyspnoea. Hyperinflated chest and low PEFR.

Differential diagnosis

The choice lies between reversible and irreversible airflow limitation, i.e. asthma and chronic obstructive airways disease. While there can be some fixed obstruction in asthma and reversibility in chronic airways disease, it is reasonable to allow the presence of **significant** reversibility to differentiate the two.

It is clear from the examination that he has a hyperinflated chest. The symptoms are entirely in keeping with either diagnosis. Indeed, part of the point of this question is to test whether or not you know that asthma can present predominantly with cough. The therapeutic interventions reported no longer help, but that does not make the differential diagnosis any easier. The dose of steroids is too low and the length of the course too short to be able to draw a conclusion of irreversibility. On the basis of the fact that the cough is dry, there is unlikely to be much disease of the bronchi and bronchioles, again limiting the type of chronic airflow limitation. However, in his thirties he had a disease that responded to bronchodilators – he had asthma. Particularly given the current inadequacy of treatment, there is no reason to postulate a second disease now. In addition, he is a non-smoker and is presenting at rather a young age for this to be chronic irreversible airflow limitation.

Investigation and therapy

If he had emphysema, gas exchange would be impaired, but not in asthma. Hence I would confirm the diagnosis with DL_{CO}. The single most effective therapeutic measure would be a prolonged course of high-dose steroids.

7.4

Accepted answers

(a) 1:5

(b) Three times at 200 J, 200 J, and 360 J respectively (400 J is acceptable for the last)

(c) Lignocaine 100 mg IV or 200 mg by ET tube
Sodium bicarbonate 50 mmol (50 ml 8.4%) IV

(d) Up to 2 min

There is some latitude in the answers, but these represent the current recommendations. It is interesting to note that bicarbonate is becoming ever less popular.

Essence

Do you know how to manage a cardiac arrest?

This is one of the few situations in which it is legitimate to ask for drug doses and details of minute by minute management. There is a 'party line', the recommendations of the European Resuscitation Council (*Resuscitation* (1992) **24**, 111–21). It is wise to commit it to memory. It is also a popular subject for the oral examination in the Membership when circulating adrenaline levels reproduce the situation of managing a cardiac arrest.

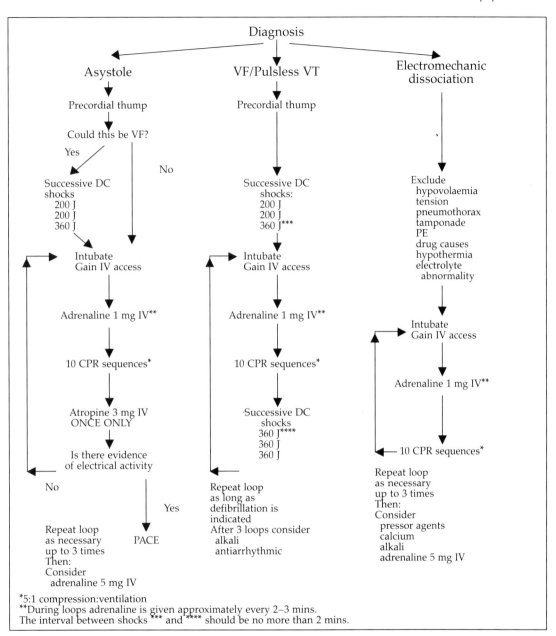

Diagnosis

Asystole / VF/Pulsless VT / Electromechanic dissociation

Asystole

Precordial thump

Could this be VF?

Yes → Successive DC shocks
200 J
200 J
360 J

No

Intubate
Gain IV access

Adrenaline 1 mg IV**

10 CPR sequences*

Atropine 3 mg IV
ONCE ONLY

Is there evidence
of electrical activity

No → Repeat loop
as necessary
up to 3 times
Then:
Consider
  adrenaline 5 mg IV

Yes → PACE

VF/Pulsless VT

Precordial thump

Successive DC shocks:
200 J
200 J
360 J***

Intubate
Gain IV access

Adrenaline 1 mg IV**

10 CPR sequences*

Successive DC shocks
360 J****
360 J
360 J

Repeat loop
as long as
defibrillation is
indicated
After 3 loops consider
  alkali
  antiarrhythmic

Electromechanic dissociation

Exclude
  hypovolaemia
  tension
  pneumothorax
  tamponade
  PE
  drug causes
  hypothermia
  electrolyte
    abnormality

Intubate
Gain IV access

Adrenaline 1 mg IV**

10 CPR sequences*

Repeat loop
as necessary
up to 3 times
Then:
Consider
  pressor agents
  calcium
  alkali
  adrenaline 5 mg IV

*5:1 compression:ventilation
**During loops adrenaline is given approximately every 2–3 mins.
The interval between shocks *** and **** should be no more than 2 mins.

7.5

Accepted answer

Neuroleptic malignant syndrome

Essence

A young schizophrenic becomes obtunded and febrile with muscle stiffness over a period of days. She has recently been to her psychiatrist.

Differential diagnosis

It would be reasonable to consider a primary psychiatric explanation for the lack of communication. But in the presence of fever and muscle stiffness it is important to exclude an organic cause, particularly since fever is a potent cause of an acute confusional state. Although infection would be the most likely cause of the fever, there are no localizing clinical features. It may be difficult to detect pneumonia or urinary tract infection clinically and encephalitis, although compatible with the fever and obtunded state, would be very unusual. There is also no reason to believe she has a deep seated infection such as endocarditis. Fevers associated with malignant and autoimmune disease are rarely this high.

We are left with the rare causes of fever, and this question relies on your recognition of a syndrome: fever, confusion and muscle stiffness over a period of days following a precipitating drug – the neuroleptic malignant syndrome (NMS).

NMS is an idiosyncratic response to phenothiazines, thioxanthines, and butyrophenones, and carries a mortality rate of up to 30%. The differential diagnosis includes encephalitis, catatonia, and malignant hyperpyrexia. The latter occurs following the use of inhalational anaesthetics and also may respond to dantrolene.

7.6

Accepted answers

(a) Vitamin B_{12} deficiency (100%)

(b) Common variable hypogammaglobulinaemia (100%)
    Common variable immunodeficiency (100%)
    Non-familial hypogammaglobulinaemia (100%)

    Lymphoma (50%)

Essence

A young man with recurrent non-bloody diarrhoea and bronchitis has splenomegaly, anaemia, lymphopenia, thrombocytopenia, hypoalbuminaemia, hypogammaglobulinaemia, gastritis, jejunal villous atrophy and mild colitis.

Differential diagnosis

You will probably choose the jejunal problem first. Does the patient have primary coeliac disease? Malabsorption might explain the hypoalbuminaemia and anaemia, but to explain the low immunoglobulin levels you would have to postulate either a protein-losing

There is a lot of information here. The first approach is to attempt to identify a syndrome. If nothing springs to mind, try to identify the single most characteristic feature. Go through the causes of that feature to determine if all the other findings fit with any single diagnosis. If that fails, choose the differential diagnosis associated with a second characteristic.

Classification of immunodeficiency*

Primary
- Antibody deficiency
  X-linked agammaglobulinaemia (Bruton)
  Non-familial hypogammaglobulinaemia
  Selective class/subclass deficiencies
  Thymoma with hypogamma-
    globulinaemia
  Transient hypogammaglobulinaemia
    (infancy)
  Transcobalamin II deficiency
- T cells
  Thymic aplasia
  Purine nucleoside phosphorylase
    deficiency
- Mixed T and B cell defects
  Severe
  Severe combined immunodeficiency
    (SCID)
    (a) unknown aetiology
    (b) adenosine deaminase deficiency
  Reticular dysgenesis
  Biotin-dependent carboxylase
    deficiencies

  Moderate
  Short limbed dwarfism and
    immunodeficiency

Orotic aciduria
Bloom's syndrome

Mild
Ataxia telangiectasia
Wiskott–Aldrich syndrome
X-linked lymphoproliferative
  syndrome

Secondary
- Antibody
  CLL
  Myeloma
  Drugs (e.g. gold, phenytoin,
    penicillamine)
  Nephrotic syndrome
  Protein-losing enteropathy
  Dystrophia myotonica
- T cell
  AIDS
  Hodgkin's disease and other
    lymphomas
  Malnutrition
  Zinc deficiency
  Drugs (e.g. steroids, cyclophosphamide,
    cyclosporin)

*After Webster, ADB, in *Oxford Textbook of Medicine*, eds. DJ Weatherall, *et al.*, second edition, OUP.

enteropathy, which is rare in coeliac disease, or malignant transformation, for which he is young. (Continue to look for a unifying diagnosis; it is better than a disease plus a complication.) Other causes of jejunal villous atrophy include infectious enteritis, lymphoma, Whipple's disease, chronic ulcerative enteritis, kwashiorkor, tropical sprue, food allergy and primary hypogammaglobulinaemia. The splenomegaly would make lymphoma high on your list, but you might have expected something more from the biopsy. Common variable hypogammaglobulinaemia is compatible with all the features of this case: presentation as a young adult (unlike other hypogamma-globulinaemias), recurrent chest infections, a coeliac-like picture and features suggestive of inflammatory bowel disease, gastritis, splenomegaly, anaemia, lymphopenia, thrombocytopenia, hypoalbuminaemia, and hypogammaglobulinaemia. Intestinal lymphangiectasia would cause hypogammaglobulinaemia, hypoalbuminaemia and lymphopenia, but is likely to have different jejunal histology. It may complicate lymphomas (which could explain his splenomegaly and anaemia) or inflammatory bowel disease (which would explain his colitis), but this would be a more complex answer. Lymphoma alone may be associated with hypogammaglobulinaemia, but the colitis and long history are strongly against it.

Answers to Case Histories Paper 8

8.1

Accepted answers

(a) Malaria – must exclude, despite atypical features (100%)
  Hepatitis A (100%) – must exclude, although rather unusual with a fever of 39.2°C at the onset of jaundice
  Hepatitis B – risk factor: homosexual; but short history (100%)
  Typhoid fever – rigors and rash atypical (100%)
  EBV (100%)
  Trypanosomiasis – hepatosplenomegaly, although not typical, is nonetheless quite often a feature (100%)
  African tick typhus fever (100%)
  Relapsing fever – rash atypical (100%)

  Typhus fever (75%) – too general a term

  Leptospirosis – unlikely without a neutrophilia (50%)
  Yellow fever – hepatosplenomegaly and lymphadenopathy not typical, and the patient has had 'all appropriate immunizations' (25%)

(b) HIV serology (100%)
  Repeated blood cultures as temperature rises (100%)

  These two investigations are essential. The remaining three are dictated by your answers in section (a), and should be as follows:
  Repeated thick and thin blood films (malaria) (100%)
  Hepatitis A serology (hepatitis A) (100%)
  Hepatitis B serology (hepatitis B) (100%)
  Faecal and urine culture (typhoid fever) (you will already have included blood culture above) (100%)
  EBV serology (EBV) (100%)
  Blood film or buffy coat (trypanosomiasis) (100%)
  Rickettsia serology (African tick typhus fever) (100%)
  Blood film for *Borrelia* spirochaetes (relapsing fever) (100%)

  Leptospira serology (leptospirosis) (50%)

  Yellow fever serology (yellow fever) (25%)

Essence

A young homosexual returning from Zambia develops a febrile illness with a rash, abdominal pain, hepatocellular jaundice, hepatosplenomegaly, and lymphadenopathy.

Differential diagnosis

In this case the number of differential diagnoses is enormous. In every ill traveller returning from the tropics you must exclude malaria, typhoid fever and yellow fever.

Antimalarial prophylaxis does not provide absolute protection, so malaria must be one of your answers. A clinical picture of rigors, macular erythematous rash, and lymphadenopathy (but not the splenomegaly) would be atypical for typhoid. It is difficult to exclude yellow fever clinically, but hepatosplenomegaly (although both organs are involved) and lymphadenopathy are not classical. Similarly, there are none of the expected features of a viral haemorrhagic fever.

The localizing features – rash, hepatic and splenic involvement, and abdominal pain – are also very common features of many tropical diseases. Your decision about the other diagnoses offered should take them into account. You should also consider the likelihood of acquisition of HIV in East Africa.

Finally, remember to match your diagnoses with the investigations, which takes up three investigations. The last two should be HIV serology and blood cultures.

Common causes of jaundice in a tropical traveller
Hepatitis
Malaria
Typhoid fever
G6PD deficiency
Thalassaemia
Sickle cell disease

Rarely:
  Yellow fever
  Leptospirosis

Causes of hepatosplenomegaly

Common causes

  Kala-azar (visceral leishmaniasis)
  Malaria (tropical splenomegaly syndrome)
  Chronic myeloid leukaemia
  Portal hypertension
  Myelofibrosis

Other causes

  Infections
    Viral
    Bacterial (tuberculosis [rarely], typhoid, brucellosis)
    Helminths (*Schistosoma mansoni* [in natives of endemic areas])
  Malignancies
    Leukaemia
    Reticulo-endothelial disorders
    Lymphoma
  Others
    Sarcoidosis
    Amyloidosis
    Glycogen storage disorders
    Haemachromatosis

8.2

Accepted answers

(a) Serum magnesium level (100%)

(b) Intact parathormone level (elevated) (100%)

(c) Anti-convulsant induced osteomalacia (100%)

    Osteomalacia secondary to vegetarianism (100%)

    Osteomalacia secondary to malabsorption (75%)
    Secondary hyperparathyroidism (75%)

    Primary hyperparathyroidism with vitamin D deficiency (50%)

    Steroid myopathy (25%)

(d) Bone biopsy (100%)

    Ultrasound or CT scanning of parathyroid glands for parathyroid adenoma (25%)
    Subtraction radioisotope scan of thyroid and parathyroid glands (25%)

Rejected answer

Creatinine kinase

Essence

A young man with Crohn's disease and epilepsy presenting initially with chronic diarrhoea, cramps in his hands and oedema has a low uncorrected calcium, with normal alkaline phosphatase. He later develops proximal myopathy and a raised alkaline phosphatase.

> The fact that an answer seems far too obvious does not of itself exclude it. It may not be obvious to everyone, and just occasionally, they do ask very easy questions. But be wary.

> Particularly in complex questions, take care to summarize all the positive findings.

Differential diagnosis

We shall first address the initial part of the question, to which question (a) applies. Although this patient's total calcium is low, there are several reasons to suspect that the ionized calcium level is normal: the diarrhoea is not offensive, which argues against malabsorption, as does the normal haemoglobin; the oedema suggests significant hypoalbuminaemia, for which the calcium would have to be corrected; and, finally, significant hypocalcaemia would provoke a rise in the alkaline phosphatase provided the parathyroids are functioning (there is no reason to postulate that the hypocalcaemia is of such acute onset that it is too early to induce increased parathyroid hormone secretion). Each of these would be rather soft evidence in a real clinical situation but in the context of this examination they are significant. On the positive side, any prolonged diarrhoea is associated with low magnesium levels and possible tetany. In summary, you are given a reasonable amount of evidence that correcting his calcium is not going to provide you with an answer. For that reason, magnesium is a better answer than albumin.

In the second part of the question, you have to appreciate the existence of a second pathology. The situation has changed, both clinically and biochemically. As always, ascribing the situation to a complicating problem is preferrable to making an additional unrelated diagnosis. The most striking feature now is the raised alkaline phosphatase. This is most likely to be of bony origin in this case. Chronic phenytoin therapy is associated with osteomalacia, as is vegetarianism. Malabsorption may cause osteomalacia, but as discussed, this is a less likely cause here. Osteomalacia is associated with secondary hyperparathyroidism where the interplay of calcium homeostatic mechanisms is able to maintain serum calcium in the normal range, at the expense of bone resorption (hence the raised alkaline phosphatase). The low (corrected) serum calcium in this case should alert you to the fact that homeostasis is breaking down: vitamin D is necessary for parathormone to have its full effect. Finally, Crohn's disease may be associated with granulomatous infiltration of the liver or with malignancy, both of which can cause a raised alkaline phosphatase. However, that is unlikely to be the explanation here.

The fact that the vitamin D level is almost normal leaves the possibility that parathormone is elevated as a primary event: the chicken rather than the egg. This is less attractive since it is not linked to pre-existing pathology, but it cannot be excluded on the basis of the information provided. Steroid myopathy remains a possibility but would score low marks as the patient's steroid-dependent disease is quiescent and the steroids are presumably now only being given in low dose, if at all.

Causes of raised alkaline phosphatase
- Bone disease
   - Osteomalacia
   - Rickets
   - Primary hyperparathyroidism (if bone disease)
   - Paget's disease (very high levels)
   - Secondary deposits
   - Primary osteogenic sarcoma
- Liver disease
   - Cholestasis
   - Hepatitis
   - Cirrhosis (but not always)
   - Malignancy
   - Granulomata
   - Hepatic congestion
- Pregnancy (third trimester)
- Children until puberty

Muscle enzymes are of no help in establishing the cause of the myopathy, not least because he has just fallen down a flight of stairs.

Bone biopsy will establish the presence of defective mineralization in osteomalacia, and will show the characteristic fibrosis of hyperparathyroidism if there is adequate vitamin D. Imaging of parathyroid adenomas is difficult, and in a simpler case referral for surgery could be made even without visualizing an adenoma, because failure to image pre-operatively does not exclude the presence of a tumour.

The nature of anticonvulsant osteomalacia is not clearly understood. It is simplest to presume that hepatic enzyme induction by anticonvulsants results in conversion of precursors to metabolites other than 25-hydroxycalciferol, but some patients have normal levels of 1,25-dihydroxycalciferol despite florid osteomalacia, suggesting a more complex mechanism.

Another moot point in this question is the nature of osteomalacia-related myopathy; muscle enzymes are often normal (unlike in the myopathy of hypothyroidism) and there is some evidence to suggest that high levels of parathormone themselves are associated with myopathy.

8.3

Accepted answers

(a) Pericardial haemorrhage due to uraemic pericarditis (100%)

Pneumothorax / haemothorax / haemo-pneumothorax following insertion of subclavian line (100%)

Pulmonary oedema due to fluid overload (75%)

Pulmonary oedema due to myocardial infarction (75%)

Pulmonary oedema (50%)

(b) Insertion of pericardial drain
Pericardiectomy
Insertion of chest drain

Rejected answer

Pulmonary haemorrhage
Pulmonary embolism

Essence

A long-standing poorly controlled diabetic with proliferative retinopathy with end-stage renal failure who deteriorates after starting dialysis.

Differential diagnosis

One possible cause of this man's deterioration is a pneumothorax or haemothorax (or both) caused by the insertion of the subclavian line. This may be a spontaneous event some hours after the insertion of the line, blood may have accumulated gradually, or a bleed may have occurred after the patient was anticoagulated for haemodialysis. Haemothorax is a marginally better answer since a pneumothorax is likely to have been picked up on chest X-ray taken to check the position of the line. Alternatively, he may have pericarditis due to chronic uraemia which, similarly, may be complicated by pericardial haemorrhage as a result of the anticoagulation.

Pulmonary oedema is a less likely explanation of his deterioration. He was fluid overloaded on admission, and certainly had pulmonary oedema; dialysis would, however, make this better, not worse. Indeed, in the

clinical situation of fluid overload it is likely that the priority would have been to remove fluid by ultrafiltration before instituting dialysis. On the other hand, he is at risk of ischaemic heart disease and, particularly on dialysis, he might suffer an acute myocardial infarction (often silent in diabetics), which itself could exacerbate the pulmonary oedema.

Pulmonary haemorrhage is a recognized complication of renal failure, but only in certain pathological states (e.g. vasculitis, SLE, Goodpasture's syndrome) and would be very unlikely in this patient.

The treatment of haemo/pneumothorax would be to insert a chest drain. Pericardial haemorrhage might need pericardiectomy, but you may need to insert a pericardial drain initially.

> It is common for two parts of a question to be linked. If, for example, you are asked to offer two investigations to confirm your two diagnoses, do not be tempted to try and sneak another diagnosis 'under the wire' by offering an unlinked investigation. In this examination you must show that you have the self-confidence to act in a consistent manner.

8.4

Accepted answers

(a) Repeat bronchoscopy with transbronchial biopsy
   CT or MRI scan of head
(b) Sarcoidosis involving CNS

Essence

A young man develops over several years two episodes of a 'flu-like illness, nodular shadows on chest X-ray, negative Kveim and Mantoux tests and later has a seizure.

Differential diagnosis

The important point about this question is to understand the limitations of special investigations. The negative Kveim test is of no help since it does not exclude sarcoidosis. Similarly, the negative brochoscopy and transbronchial biopsy are of no help. We know from the radiography that there is an abnormality. The failure to respond to a reducing course of steroids is a rather useless piece of information; it is only of diagnostic value if you know how much was given for how long and the nature of the follow-up.

Of more interest is the negative Mantoux test. If he had tuberculosis one would expect this man to be much worse in order to be anergic to PPD. Similarly one would expect most British people to be positive to a Mantoux of 1:1000. This fact, coupled with relatively asymptomatic pulmonary disease, and subsequent CNS involvement produces a syndrome that is really only compatible with sarcoidosis.

The two investigations of choice would be an MRI or CT scan to identify the CNS lesions, and a repeat transbronchial biopsy to try and obtain a tissue diagnosis. It would be inappropriately invasive to proceed to an open lung biopsy before trying another bronchoscopy, and it would be unreasonable, in the face of such a striking clinical syndrome, to subject him to an open operation for the purpose of obtaining tissue from what is probably now rather a chronic scarred lesion.

8.5

Accepted answer

'Ecstasy' abuse
3,4-methylenedioxymethamphetamine (MDMA) abuse

Essence

A young man is found unconscious having been well 4 h earlier. He is shocked, hyperpyrexial and has fixed pupils.

Differential diagnosis

There are very few reasons for a young man suddenly becoming this ill. This is not a picture of diabetes. (You do not even need the

blood glucose to tell you that.) The only infective diseases which would make someone this ill are septicaemia, meningitis or encephalitis. The temperature is too high for a normal bacterial infection and he is unlikely to be shocked if he has a viral infection. A patient with profound immunosuppression could become this ill very quickly, but it would be extremely unusual for this to be the initial presentation of a myeloproliferative or lymphoproliferative disease or AIDS. The orofacial dyskinesia is known as 'bruxism'.

The most likely acute insult in this case is substance abuse and the picture is typical of the severe effects of 3,4-methylenedioxymethamphetamine (MDMA) or 'ecstasy' – or just 'E'. No other substance is likely to cause this syndrome. In fact this patient had taken three tablets and died a few hours after admission.

No other diagnosis fits as well. Malignant hyperthermia follows anaesthetic agents. Neuroleptic malignant syndrome is associated with muscle stiffness and there is no history of psychiatric illness. Cocaine would cause small pupils.

> **Causes of hyperpyrexia**
> - Infection
> - Heatstroke
> - Cerebrovascular accident
> - Neuroleptic malignant syndrome
> - Malignant hyperthermia
> - Monoamine oxidase inhibitor overdose
> - Substance abuse
>   'Ecstasy'
>   Amphetamine
>   Metamphetamine
>   Cocaine

8.6

Accepted answers

Factor IX deficiency
Haemophilia B

Essence

A 6-year-old boy presents with a painful, red, swollen knee. There is no evidence of systemic infection but he has a prolonged APTT with normal factor VIII levels

Differential diagnosis

The clinical history suggests a differential diagnosis of haemarthrosis or septic arthritis.

However, the prolonged APTT make this a haemarthrosis. The normal bleeding time and platelet level make this a defect of the clotting cascade, and the APTT and prothrombin time put it in the intrinsic pathway. The most common defect, factor VIII deficiency or haemophilia A, is excluded; the answer is the next most likely, factor IX deficiency or haemophilia B. The lack of a family history is of no significance as one-third of patients carry new mutations.

SECTION 2

SECTION 2 – DATA INTERPRETATION

In many ways the data interpretation section is the easiest for which to prepare since you can only be asked about a finite number of medical investigations. Although it would be too much for a candidate to be familiar with them all, it does mean you can have a fair idea of the sort of data you are going to be shown.

If we take cardiology as an example, it is almost certain that you will be asked to interpret an ECG, whereas it is less likely that you will be shown an echocardiogram. Going one step further, the ECG, which is a very common investigation, may well be difficult to interpret. On the other hand the echocardiogram, a more specialist investigation, will probably show one of only a few cardiac abnormalities. In other words, expect difficult examples of common investigations and more straightforward examples of specialist investigations.

The lessons from this should be obvious. In preparation for the examination:

- Take each speciality at a time and try to predict the investigations about which you might be questioned.
- For the more common investigations, practise a logical, reproducible approach to the data which will help you arrive at the correct diagnosis – much as you are taught to examine the various components of the ECG one at a time.
- For the less common investigations, try to construct short lists of the conditions likely to be represented. In the examination, if you are having difficulty reaching a diagnosis, run these through your mind to see which fits best. In this book, we shall try to provide you with a list of the most likely diagnoses for most of these specialist investigations.

As you work your way through the following papers, we will try to develop these principles for specific sets of data.

The advice we gave before the case histories section also applies here: as you turn over the examination paper, prepare a timetable based on the number of questions and keep to it. Miss out questions that you find difficult and remember to write neat, precise and full answers.

Now start working your way through the following papers. Try to work under examination conditions, timing yourself and resisting the temptation to look at the answers before you have finished. At the beginning of each paper, check how many questions there are and divide all but the last ten minutes equally amongst them. Be strict with yourself in keeping to those times. Write down your answers as you will write them in the examination. If you do not, then you will take undue comfort from having thought of the right answer during consideration of a question, even if it was not your final answer.

Data Interpretation Paper 1

1.1

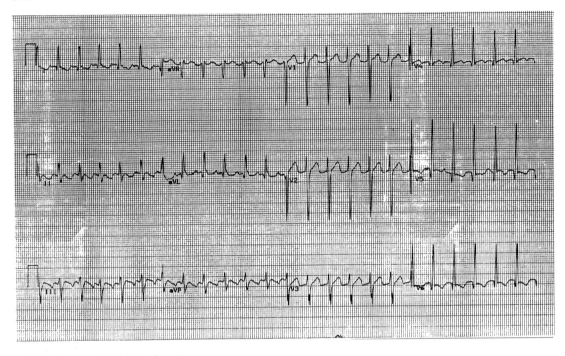

(a) What does this ECG show?
(b) How might you confirm this?

1.2

A 37-year-old woman presents with weight gain, amenorrhoea and hypertension.
Investigations show:

Plasma sodium	138 mmol/l
Plasma potassium	2.7 mmol/l
Plasma cortisol at 9 a.m.	840 nmol/l *(normal range 280–700)*
Plasma cortisol at 9 a.m. following 2 mg dexamethasone 6-hourly for 2 days	150 nmol/l

(a) What is the likely diagnosis?
(b) Give two reasons for the hypokalaemia.
(c) Give two useful radiological investigations.
(d) What therapy would you recommend?
(e) Give one common endocrine complication of therapy.

1.3

A 25-year-old man was brought in to Casualty at 2 a.m. smelling of alcohol. The following results were obtained:

Plasma sodium	133 mmol/l
Plasma potassium	6.9 mmol/l
Plasma urea	22 mmol/l
Plasma creatinine	2254 μmol/l
Plasma calcium	1.87 mmol/l
Plasma phosphate	1.99 mmol/l

What is the cause of his renal impairment?

1.4

A healthy 33-year-old female patient asks your advice concerning cystic fibrosis. She had an 18-year-old brother who died of the disease. The patient and her two sisters, both of whom are also in their thirties, are unaffected. A younger brother died at the age of 5 in a road traffic accident.

As she is planning to get married and start a family, she wishes to know the probability of her own children developing the disease. Assuming the frequency of the cystic fibrosis gene in the general population is 1/25, what is that probability? The patient is unrelated to her future husband.

1.5

A 50-year-old former shipyard worker complained of breathlessness. Respiratory function tests were performed:

	Predicted	*Actual*
FEV$_1$ (l)	4.1	3.9
FVC (l)	5.0	2.6
TL$_{CO}$ (mmol/min/kPa)	10.2	6.6
K$_{CO}$ (mmol/min/kPa/l)	1.9	2.1

(a) What defect in respiratory function do these results show?
(b) What is the probable diagnosis?

1.6

The following data were obtained at cardiac catheterization:

Site	Oxygen saturation (%)
Superior vena cava	72
Inferior vena cava	76
Right atrium	75
Right ventricle	84
Pulmonary artery	85
Left ventricle	98
Aorta	97

What is the diagnosis?

1.7

A 25-year-old mechanic presents with apathy and tremor. Urinalysis shows glycosuria. The blood chemistry showed:

Plasma sodium	140 mmol/l
Plasma potassium	3.0 mmol/l
Plasma glucose	4.8 mmol/l
Plasma bicarbonate	14 mmol/l
Plasma aspartate aminotransferase	55 IU/l *(normal range 5–35)*
Plasma bilirubin	31 μmol/l

(a) What is the diagnosis?
(b) Give two investigations to confirm the diagnosis.
(c) Suggest two other physical signs which may be present.

1.8

A 29-year-old Iraqi postgraduate student gives a 3-month history of weight loss, malaise and night sweats. He has pallor, abdominal distention and hepatosplenomegaly.
   Investigations:

Hb	7.8 g/dl
MCV	80 fl
Wbc	2.1×10^9/l
	68% lymphocytes
Platelets	82×10^9/l
Blood film	normocytic normochromic anaemia
ESR	72 mm in 1st hour
Plasma calcium	2.48 mmol/l
	contd

Plasma aspartate aminotransferase	72 IU/l *(normal range 5–35)*
Plasma alkaline phosphatase	112 IU/l *(normal range 30–100)*
Serum albumin	24 g/l
Serum globulin	64 g/l
Chest X-ray	normal

(a) Give two possible diagnoses.
(b) Name two investigations which you would request to make a diagnosis.

1.9

The 5-year-old son of working-class parents has become lethargic and irritable. His mother has noticed that he stumbles.
 The cerebrospinal fluid examination was clear with an opening pressure of 300 mm.

CSF:	White cells	$3/mm^3$
	Protein	2.1 g/l
	Glucose	4 mmol/l
Plasma glucose		6 mmol/l

(a) What is the most likely diagnosis?
(b) What simple investigation would you order next?

1.10

The effects of a new antihypertensive drug were tested on a group of patients. The effect of the drug after 3 months was assessed by comparing the mean arterial pressures of control and treated groups using Student's t test.
 The value of p was 0.01.

(a) What was the null hypothesis?
(b) What form of distribution does this analysis assume about the blood pressures within the study populations?
(c) What is the probability that the difference between the two groups was due to chance?

Data Interpretation Paper 2

2.1

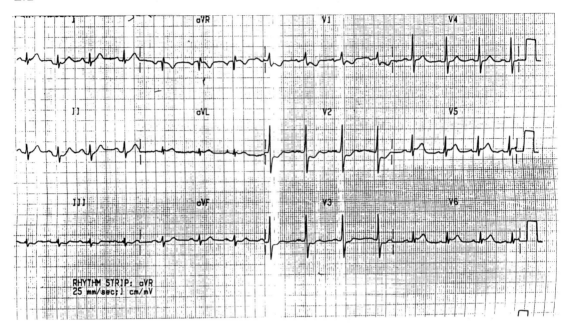

This is the ECG of a 60-year-old man who presents with chest pain.

What is the diagnosis?

2.2

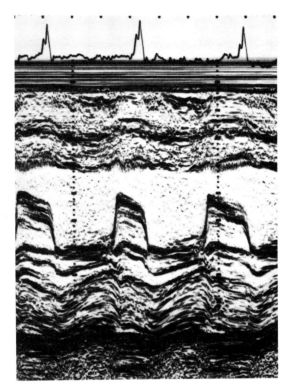

This M-mode echocardiogram is from a 63-year-old woman who is breathless on exertion.

What is the diagnosis?

2.3

A 65-year-old tramp who frequently visits the Accident and Emergency department is proving more difficult to eject than normal. He is noted to have widespread lymphadenopathy.
Haematological examination:

Hb	8.9 g/dl
Wbc	123×10^9/l
Platelets	195×10^9/l
MCV	109 fl

(a) What is the most likely cause of the elevated white cell count?
(b) Give three reasons for the elevated MCV.

2.4

A 30-year-old Turkish Cypriot waiter presents with fever, diarrhoea, abdominal pain, weight loss and arthritis. He has had several similar episodes in the past. On examination, he is thin with clinical evidence of a small left pleural effusion and marked ankle oedema.

Investigations show:

Hb	13.2 g/dl
MCV	101.3 fl
Serum albumin	25 g/l
Faecal fat	85 mmol/24 h
	(normal range 11–18 mmol/l)
Urinary xylose excretion after 25 g oral load	3.2 mmol/5 h
	(normal range 8.0–16.0/24 h)
Urinalysis	protein + + +

(a) What is the diagnosis?
(b) What diagnostic test would you perform?
(c) What treatment would you consider?
(d) What is the cause of the pleural effusion?

2.5

A 48-year-old pilot becomes acutely short of breath.
  Arterial blood gas analysis shows:

pH	7.38
PaO_2	8.0 kPa
$PaCO_2$	3.6 kPa

(a) What is the likely diagnosis?
(b) Suggest four other possible diagnoses.

2.6

A 56-year-old man presents with a 6-month history of back pain and recent nausea and vomiting. He is now anuric.
  Investigations show:

Plasma sodium	146 mmol/l
Plasma potassium	5.7 mmol/l
Plasma urea	56 mmol/l
Plasma creatinine	1020 μmol/l
Plasma calcium	2.95 mmol/l
Plasma phosphate	1.1 mmol/l
Serum total protein	96 g/dl
Serum albumin	32 g/dl
Hb	9.4 g/dl

(a) What is the diagnosis?
(b) List three investigations which would help confirm this.

2.7

A GP asks for your advice. He has just received a copy of these investigations, performed in the out-patient department on a patient who had recently presented with hypertension and peripheral oedema.

Investigations show:

Plasma sodium	137 mmol/l
Plasma potassium	8.9 mmol/l
Plasma urea	13.8 mmol/l
Plasma creatinine	210 μmol/l
Plasma calcium	2.1 mmol/l
Plasma phosphate	3.9 mmol/l
Plasma glucose	1.5 mmol/l

What is the most likely cause of the abnormalities?

2.8

A 38-year-old secretary gives a 9-month history of generalized pruritus and intermittent, pale, foul-smelling stools. On examination, she is icteric and has spider naevi.

Investigations show:

Hb	11.6 g/dl
Wbc	8.0×10^9/l
Plasma bilirubin	40 μmol/l
Plasma aspartate aminotransferase	90 IU/l *(normal range 5–35)*
Plasma alkaline phosphatase	350 IU/l *(normal range 30–100)*
Serum albumin	34 g/l
Serum globulin	48 g/l
Plasma cholesterol	9.0 mmol/l
Hepatitis B surface antigen	negative
Antinuclear factor	negative
Anti-Sm antibodies	positive

(a) What is the most likely diagnosis?
(b) Suggest two other investigations which would confirm the diagnosis.

2.9

A 19-year-old man complains that his feet feel numb. Neurophysiological studies show the following:

Sural sensory action potential	6 μV *(normal > 15 μV)*
Median nerve sensory action potential	4 μV *(normal > 20 μV)*
Common peroneal nerve motor conduction velocity	47 m/s *(normal > 45 m/s)*

(a) What is the pathological basis of the numbness?
(b) Suggest two possible diagnoses.

2.10

A 46-year-old woman complains of muscle aches and weakness. On examination she has a rash on her face and on the dorsum of her hands. Telangiectasia are present on her face. There is no significant family history.
   Investigations show:

Plasma sodium	141 mmol/l
Plasma potassium	4.1 mmol/l
Plasma urea	5.0 mmol/l
Plasma calcium	2.90 mmol/l
Plasma aspartate aminotransferase	15 IU/l *(normal range 5–35)*
Plasma creatine phosphokinase	820 IU/l *(normal range 25–170)*
Hb	10.9 g/dl
Wbc	6.0 $\times$ 10^9/l
ESR	46 mm in 1st hour

(a) What is the most likely diagnosis?
(b) Give one important association found with this disorder.

Data Interpretation Paper 3

3.1

A heart murmur is investigated by cardiac catheterization.

Site	Pressure (mmHg)	Oxygen saturation (%)
Superior vena cava		60
Inferior vena cava		66
Right atrium (mean pressure)	5	88
Right ventricle	60/5	90
Pulmonary artery	15/4	89
Pulmonary wedge (mean pressure)	6	

(a) Give two abnormalities.
(b) Give two conditions which give rise to these in combination.

3.2

This is the ECG of a 38-year-old unconscious male.

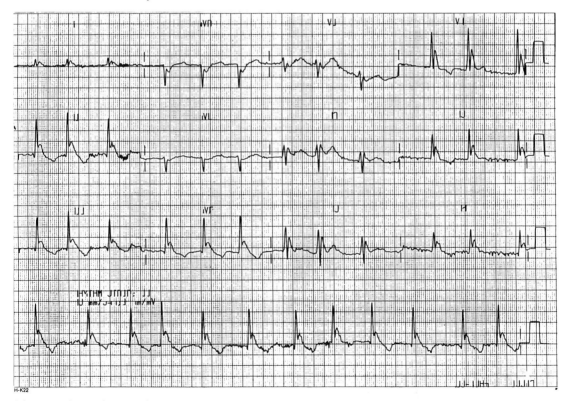

(a) Give three abnormalities.
(b) What is the diagnosis?

3.3

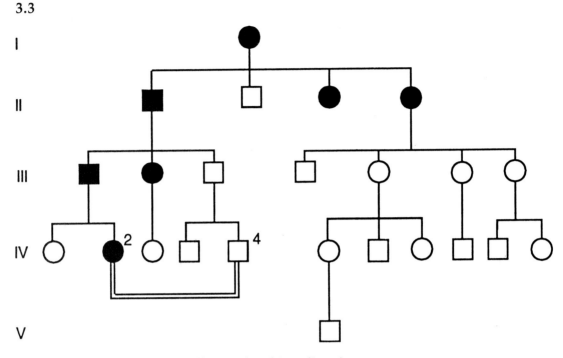

(a) What mode of inheritance is illustrated in this pedigree?
(b) What is the probability of an affected offspring resulting from the marriage of IV^2 and IV^4?

3.4

A 24-year-old man with progressive low back pain and weakness finally sees his doctor with an episode of left loin pain. Investigations show haematuria and a urinary pH of 7.
  Other investigations show:

Plasma sodium	135 mmol/l
Plasma potassium	2.8 mmol/l
Plasma urea	5.7 mmol/l
Plasma creatinine	107 μmol/l
Plasma chloride	115 mmol/l
Plasma bicarbonate	16 mmol/l

(a) What is the diagnosis?
(b) Suggest two abnormalities which might be seen on a plain abdominal X-ray.
(c) What is the cause of his back pain?

3.5

A 15-year-old girl presents with breathlessness. Blood gas analysis shows:

pH	7.49
PCO_2	6.4 kPa
PO_2	4.8 kPa
Plasma bicarbonate	15 mmol/l

What is your next investigation?

3.6

An 18-year-old unmarried female presents with heavy bleeding per vagina. She is febrile and admits to 2 months of amenorrhoea prior to this episode.
    Investigations show:

Hb	6.2 g/dl
Wbc	$24 \times 10^9/l$
Platelets	$30 \times 10^9/l$
Prothrombin time	31 s *(control 12 s)*
Activated partial thromboplastin time	60 s *(control 32 s)*
Fibrinogen degradation products	400 mg/l *(normal < 100 mg/l)*

(a) What important haematological information is missing?
(b) Give two pathological conditions present.
(c) Give two possible aetiologies.

3.7

A 39-year-old male with a history of rhinitis develops asthma and a purpuric rash. Results of investigations are as follows:

Hb	11.9 g/dl
MCV	93 fl
MCH	31 pg
Wbc	$10.0 \times 10^9/l$
Neutrophils	$4.6 \times 10^9/l$
Eosinophils	$1.9 \times 10^9/l$
Basophils	$0.04 \times 10^9/l$
Monocytes	$0.6 \times 10^9/l$
Lymphocytes	$2.9 \times 10^9/l$
Platelets	$239 \times 10^9/l$
ESR	45 mm in first hour

contd

Plasma sodium   144 mmol/l
Plasma potassium   4.1 mmol/l
Plasma urea   5.1 mmol/l
Anti-neutrophil cytoplasmic antibody detected
    perinuclear pattern of staining ethanol-fixed neutrophils
Anti-myeloperoxidase antibody detected
Urinalysis   no abnormality detected
Chest X-ray   several patchy shadows in both lung fields

What is the diagnosis?

3.8

A 23-year-old medical student complains of lethargy, cough and intermittent headache of 4 weeks' duration. He has mild neck stiffness but no focal neurological signs.
    CSF findings:

Opening pressure   270 mm
Appearance   straw coloured
Fluid:
    Cells 205×10^6/l (205/mm^3)
                       (88% lymphocytes, 8% neutrophils, 4% neutrophils)
    Protein   1.2 g/l
    Glucose   1.4 mmol/l
Plasma glucose   5.4 mmol/l
VDRL   negative
Indian ink stain   negative

(a) What is the most likely diagnosis?
(b) Give two initial investigations you would perform to help confirm the diagnosis.

3.9

A 27-year-old married woman with amenorrhoea of 7 months' duration is found to have mild jaundice, hepatosplenomegaly, lymphadenopathy and palmar erythema.
    Investigations show:

Hb   10.4 g/dl
Wbc 2.8×10^9/l
Platelets 72×10^9/l
ESR   29 mm in 1st hour
Plasma bilirubin   58 μmol/l
Plasma aspartate aminotransferase   190 IU/l
                                      (normal range 5–35)
Plasma alanine aminotransferase   105 IU/l
                                      (normal range 5–35)
                                      contd

Plasma alkaline phosphatase	65 IU/l
	(normal range 30–100)
Serum albumin	35 g/l
Serum globulin	68 g/l
Hepatitis B surface antigen	negative
Antinuclear factor	positive at titre of 1/512
Anti-Sm antibodies	positive
Anti-mitochondrial antibodies	positive at titre of 1/64

(a) What is the diagnosis?
(b) List two possible aetiologies.

3.10

A 27-year-old Jamaican female student presents with a 3-week history of fever, polyarthralgia, and a facial skin rash. She also has cervical and axillary lymphadenopathy.
    Investigations show:

Plasma calcium	2.45 mmol/l
Plasma aspartate aminotransferase	18 IU/l
	(normal range 5–35)
Plasma alanine aminotransferase	18 IU/l
	(normal range 5–35)
Plasma alkaline phosphatase	40 IU/l
	(normal range 30–100)
Serum globulin	58 g/l
Hb	9.9 g/dl
Wbc	7.2×10^9/l
ESR	43 mm in 1st hour
C-reactive protein	6 mg/l
	(normal < 5)
VDRL	positive
TPHA	negative
Anti-nuclear factor	positive

(a) What is the likely diagnosis?
(b) Suggest one test which would strengthen the diagnosis.
(c) List three central nervous system complications of this disease.

Data Interpretation Paper 4

4.1

A 56-year-old woman presents with dyspnoea. An echocardiogram is performed.

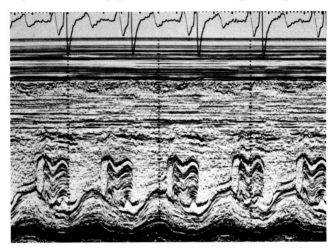

What is the diagnosis?

4.2

Following a routine insurance medical, a 32-year-old man is referred for investigation of a raised bilirubin.

Investigations show:

Plasma sodium	140 mmol/l
Plasma potassium	4.2 mmol/l
Plasma urea	5.2 mmol/l
Plasma bilirubin	37 mmol/l
Plasma alkaline phosphatase	81 IU/l *(normal range 30–100)*
Plasma aspartate aminotransferase	30 IU/l *(normal range 5–35)*
Serum albumin	41 g/l
Urinalysis	no abnormality

(a) What is the most likely diagnosis?
(b) What treatment would you advise?

4.3

A 43-year-old woman presents with a 2-month history of nausea and pruritis. The following investigations are performed:

Plasma sodium	142 mmol/l
Plasma potassium	5.9 mmol/l
Plasma urea	36.9 mmol/l
Plasma creatinine	1152 μmol/l
Hb	7.9 g/dl
MCV	58 fl
Serum ferritin	120 μmol/l
	(normal range 15–300)

(a) Give two causes of this women's anaemia.
(b) What additional test would you request?

4.4

A 36-year-old woman presents with a 2-week history of haemoptysis and a 5-day history of haematuria. In the last 24 h she has become increasingly dyspnoeic and oliguric.
   Investigations show:

Plasma sodium	136 mmol/l
Plasma potassium	8.9 mmol/l
Plasma bicarbonate	14 mmol/l
Plasma urea	48 mmol/l
Plasma creatinine	987 μmol/l
Hb	10 g/dl
Chest X-ray	patchy interstitial infiltrate

(a) What is the most likely diagnosis?
(b) Give two investigations which would confirm this.
(c) Give two other possible diagnoses.

4.5

A 72-year-old man presents with a history of pain in his right leg.
   Investigations show:

Plasma sodium	141 mmol/l
Plasma potassium	4.2 mmol/l
Plasma bicarbonate	24 mmol/l
Plasma urea	6 mmol/l
Plasma creatinine	90 μmol/l
Plasma calcium	2.45 mmol/l
	contd

Plasma phosphate	1.3 mmol/l
Serum bilirubin	12 μmol/l
Serum albumin	50 g/l
Plasma alkaline phosphatase	1364 IU/l *(normal range 30–100)*
Plasma aspartate aminotransferase	18 IU/l *(normal range 5–35)*

(a) What is the diagnosis?
(b) How would you confirm this?
(c) What is the initial treatment?

4.6

A 28-year-old woman has been on carbimazole for 1 year. She has recently noticed that her menses have become less frequent and shorter. She is attempting to divorce her husband, and appears anxious, with sweaty palms.

Thyroid function tests show the following:

| Thyroxine | 75 nmol/l *(normal 50–150)* |
| TSH | 0.2 mU/l *(normal 0.5–5)* |

(a) What is the diagnosis?
(b) What test would you do to confirm this?
(c) What is the definitive treatment?

4.7

A 23-year-old man returns from a holiday in the United States with a skin rash. He complains of a drooping right eyelid.

CSF examination reveals clear fluid with an opening pressure of 16 cm.

Fluid analysis:

Protein	1.5 g/l
White cells	56/mm^3 (80% lymphocytes)
Glucose	2.0 mmol/l
Plasma glucose	5 mmol/l

(a) What is the likely diagnosis?
(b) What investigation would confirm it?

4.8

A 22-year-old woman develops dyspnoea and chest pain after an argument with her husband's mistress. She has tachypnoea and tetany on admission and is given 35% oxygen in casualty.
    Investigations show:

Plasma sodium	139 mmol/l
Plasma potassium	4.2 mmol/l
Plasma calcium	2.22 mmol/l
Plasma glucose	4.6 mmol/l
Hb	12.8 g/dl
Wbc	6.1×10^9/l
Arterial blood gases	
pH	7.58
$PaCO_2$	2.9 kPa
PaO_2	18 kPa
HCO_3^-	19 mmol/l
Base excess	12 mmol/l
Chest X-ray	normal

(a) Describe the acid–base abnormality.
(b) What is the diagnosis?
(c) What is your immediate treatment?

4.9

This is an audiogram of a left-handed gamekeeper who complained of hearing loss. There is no air-bone gap.

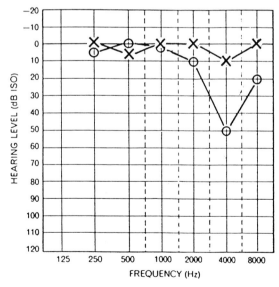

O – right
X – left

(a) What does it demonstrate?
(b) What is the likely aetiology?

4.10

A 53-year-old woman was investigated for a 6-month history of low back pain. Investigations showed:

Plasma sodium	136 mmol/l
Plasma potassium	4.2 mmol/l
Plasma urea	5.7 mmol/l
Plasma creatinine	98 μmol/l
Serum bilirubin	36 μmol/l
Serum albumin	42 g/l
Plasma aspartate aminotransferase	16 IU/l *(normal range 5–35)*
Plasma alkaline phosphatase	78 IU/l *(normal range 30–100)*
Serum IgG	28.5 g/l *(normal range 7.2–19)*
Serum IgA	2.3 g/l *(normal range 0.85–5)*
Serum IgM	2.0 g/l *(normal range 0.5–2)*
Hb	13.5 g/dl
Wbc	5.9×10^9/l
Platelets	187×10^9/l
ESR	49 mm in the first hour
Serum electrophoresis	IgG λ paraprotein band paraprotein concentration 18 g/l
Urine electrophoresis	no protein
Radiological skeletal survey	no abnormality

(a) What is the diagnosis?
(b) What further investigation would help confirm this?
(c) What course of action would you recommend?

Data Interpretation Paper 5

5.1

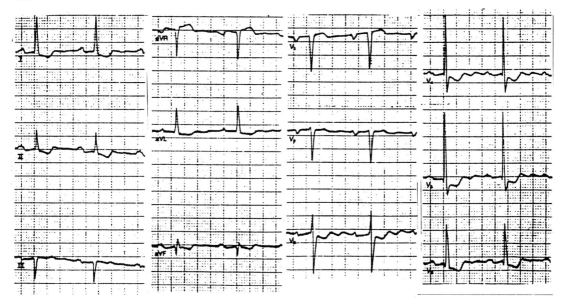

(a) Give four abnormalities present on this ECG.
(b) Suggest a cause.

5.2

Following an acute myocardial infarction, a 55-year-old man presents with mild dyspnoea and ankle swelling. When there is no response to diuretics, a pulmonary flotation catheter is used to obtain the following pressures:

Site	Pressure (mmHg)
Right atrium (mean)	6
Right ventricle	22/10
Pulmonary artery	19/8
Pulmonary wedge (mean)	4

What is the diagnosis?

5.3

A 27-year-old female patient approaches you for advice. She has an only child, a 10-year-old boy, with an autosomal recessive disease. Her husband (the boy's father) died several years ago, but your patient has since married a cousin on her mother's side of the family. She wishes to know whether a child resulting from her new marriage will also have the disease.

What is the probability of this occurring?

5.4

A 28-year-old male presents with an itchy vesicular rash on his buttocks and a 4-month history of intermittent, foul-smelling, liquid stools and weight loss.
  Investigations show:

Hb	7.9 g/dl
Wbc	6×10^9/l
MCV	105 fl
MCHC	30 g/dl
ESR	14 mm in 1st hour
Blood film	macrocytosis and microcytosis
Serum iron	8 mmol/l
	(normal range 13–22)
Serum albumin	27 g/l
Serum globulin	40 g/l
Plasma aspartate aminotransferase	18 IU/l
	(normal range 5–35)
Plasma alkaline phosphatase	40 IU/l
	(normal range 30–100)

(a) What is the rash?
(b) What is the most likely diagnosis?
(c) What test would confirm the diagnosis?

5.5

A 68-year-old woman with rheumatoid arthritis has had two recent episodes of pneumonia.
  Investigations show:

Hb	10.1 g/dl
MCV	89 fl
Wbc	1.7×10^9/l
Neutrophils	0.6×10^9/l
Platelets	53×10^9/l

(a) What is the most likely diagnosis?
(b) What physical sign would you be keen to elicit?

5.6

A 65-year-old woman complains of proximal muscle weakness. Investigations show the following:

Plasma sodium	130 mmol/l
Plasma potassium	4.2 mmol/l
Serum creatine phosphokinase	740 IU/l *(normal range 25–170)*
Hb	12.1 g/dl
MCV	102 fl

(a) What is the diagnosis?
(b) Suggest three other signs she may have.
(c) Suggest three useful investigations.

5.7

Two weeks following an episode of diarrhoea, a 27-year-old man presents acutely unwell.
    Investigations show:

Plasma sodium	143 mmol/l
Plasma potassium	8.5 mmol/l
Plasma bicarbonate	12 mmol/l
Plasma urea	53 mmol/l
Plasma creatinine	1231 μmol/l
Hb	7 g/dl
Wbc	7.6×10^9/l
Platelets	15×10^9/l

(a) What is the most likely diagnosis?
(b) Give two abnormalities you would expect to see on the blood film.

5.8

A 45-year-old farmer with a long history of hay fever developed an intermittent dry cough.
    Respiratory function tests results were as follows:

	Predicted	Actual	After bronchodilators
FEV_1 (l)	2.7	1.4	2.2
FVC (l)	3.6	2.6	3.2
FEV_1/FVC	75%	54%	
TL_{CO} (mmol/min/kPa)	8.9	8.1	
K_{CO} (mmol/min/kPa/l)	1.4	1.7	

(a) What is the respiratory abnormality?
(b) What is the likely diagnosis?

5.9

A 24-year-old woman presented to her general practitioner with influenza-like symptoms. She was prescribed amoxycillin. Two weeks later she is suffering from headaches and has vomited several times.

A lumbar puncture is performed.

CSF analysis:
Protein	1.1 g/l
Cells	80/mm^3
	(50% lymphocytes)
Glucose	6 mmol/l

No organisms seen on Gram stain and no growth on culture
Plasma glucose   20 mmol/l

(a) Give four possible diagnoses.
(b) Give three further investigations that may usefully be performed on this patient's CSF.

5.10

A 59-year-old man with a history of angina is admitted to hospital for investigation of intermittent claudication. He has a history of hypertension for which he was initially prescribed a thiazide diuretic. Six months ago this was changed to a calcium antagonist. On the surgical ward his blood pressure is consistently around 200/110 mmHg. He has a trace of ankle oedema.

Investigations show:

Plasma sodium	137 mmol/l
Plasma potassium	2.7 mmol/l
Plasma urea	8.9 mmol/l
Plasma creatinine	221 μmol/l
Hb	11.9 g/dl
Wbc	8.9×10^9/l
Platelets	388×10^9/l

What is the most likely underlying diagnosis?

Data Interpretation Paper 6

6.1

A 62-year-old woman deteriorates following emergency abdominal surgery for a perforated bowel. She is confused, hypotensive and dyspnoeic. She is transferred to the intensive therapy unit, where the following results are obtained:

Site	Pressure (mmHg)
Radial artery pressure	80/40
Right atrial pressure (mean)	6
Pulmonary artery pressure	20/8
Pulmonary capillary wedge pressure (mean)	10

Cardiac index	8.7 l/min/m² *(normal range 2.6–4.2)*
Chest X-ray	no abnormality

(a) What is the most likely diagnosis?
(b) What is the cause of her dyspnoea?

6.2

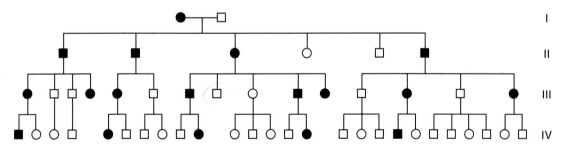

(a) Give two possible modes of inheritance.
(b) What is the probability of a son of individual III^8 inheriting the disease?

6.3

A 58-year-old Asian male alcoholic, who had been resident in the UK for the past 18 years, presented with a 3-month history of myalgia, low back pain and difficulty in walking.
   Investigations showed:

Fasting plasma glucose	3.8 mmol/l
Plasma calcium	2.10 mmol/l
Plasma phosphate	0.48 mmol/l
	contd

Serum albumin	34 g/l
Plasma aspartate aminotransferase	44 IU/l *(normal range 5–35)*
Plasma alkaline phosphatase	220 IU/l *(normal range 30–100)*
Hb	10.8 g/dl
Wbc	7.2×10^9/l
MCV	102 fl
ESR	12 mm in 1st hour

(a) What is the likely cause for his gait symptoms?
(b) List two possible causes of his macrocytic anaemia.
(c) What two treatments would you prescribe?

6.4

A 2-week-old baby presents with snuffles, skin rash and hepatomegaly. The VDRL is positive.

(a) What is the most likely diagnosis?
(b) What investigation will you request to confirm the diagnosis?

6.5

A 30-year-old man at presentation has occasional diarrhoea, a blood pressure of 200/80 mmHg and a small goitre. The results of blood tests are as follows:

Plasma sodium	139 mmol/l
Plasma potassium	4.8 mmol/l
Plasma urea	5.3 mmol/l
Plasma calcium	2.8 mmol/l
Plasma thyroxine	105 nmol/l *(normal range 50–150)*
Plasma TSH	4 mU/l *(normal range 0.5–5)*

(a) What is the diagnosis?
(b) What blood test would you order?
(c) Give two reasons for the diarrhoea.
(d) Give two reasons for the elevated calcium level.

6.6

The following data summarize the immunological data on three patients awaiting renal transplantation and one donor.

	Patient 1 (GG)	Patient 2 (RA)	Patient 3 (FG)	Donor
Age	19	44	39	32
Sex	F	M	F	M
Cause of renal failure	Anti-GBM disease	Diabetic nephropathy	Polycystic kidney disease	–
Blood group	B$^+$	B$^+$	A$^+$	B$^+$
HLA type	A2, 30	A1	A2, 29	A1, 2
	B8, 40	B8, 17	B12, 22	B12, 35
	Cw7	Cw6, 7	Cw3	Cw4
	DR3, 6	DR3, 4	DR7, 13	DR3, 11
	DRw52	DRw52	DRw52	DRw52
	DQw1, 2	DQw2, 8	DQw5, 7	DQw2, 7
Cross match with donor cells	+	–	Not tested	
Previous failed transplant				
Blood group		B$^-$		
HLA type		A1, 2		
		B8, 44		
		DR3, 4		

(a) Based on this information, which of these three patients would be the most appropriate recipient of this kidney?
(b) Give a potential disadvantage of this patient receiving the kidney.
(c) Give one reason for discarding each of the two other patients.
(d) Suggest two reasons why patient 1 may have a positive crossmatch.

6.7

A 72-year-old woman is admitted to casualty because of increasing drowsiness.
    Investigations show:

Plasma sodium	158 mmol/l
Plasma potassium	3.9 mmol/l
Plasma urea	28 mmol/l
Plasma creatinine	158 μmol/l
Plasma glucose	62 mmol/l
Arterial blood gases	
pH	7.32
PaO$_2$	11.8 kPa
PaCO$_2$	5.3 kPa
Plasma bicarbonate	19 mmol/l

(a) What is the diagnosis?
(b) Give three important steps in the management of this patient.

6.8

An 18-year-old girl is investigated because of recurrent warts, resistant to conventional treatment.
   Investigations show:

Plasma sodium	139 mmol/l
Plasma potassium	4.7 mmol/l
Plasma urea	6.3 mmol/l
Plasma creatinine	87 μmol/l
Serum bilirubin	18 μmol/l
Plasma aspartate aminotransferase	19 IU/l *(normal range 5–35)*
Plasma alkaline phosphatase	89 IU/l *(normal range 30–100)*
Serum albumin	28 g/l
Serum IgG	3.95 g/l *(normal range 7.2–19)*
Serum IgA	1.1 g/l *(normal range 0.85–5)*
Serum IgM	0.49 g/l *(normal range 0.5–2)*
Hb	12.8 g/dl
Platelets	187×10^9/l
Wbc	4.8×10^9/l
Neutrophils	3.5×10^9/l
Lymphocytes	0.9×10^9/l
Urinalysis	no abnormality

(a) What is the likely diagnosis?
(b) Suggest three investigations which might help confirm this.

6.9

A 28-year-old industrial worker presents to casualty with a 2-day history of abdominal pain, nausea and vomiting. His past medical history is unremarkable apart from intermittent high alcohol consumption.
   Investigations show:

Plasma sodium	138 mmol/l
Plasma potassium	5.1 mmol/l
Plasma urea	18.3 mmol/l
Plasma creatinine	392 μmol/l
Plasma calcium	2.3 mmol/l
Plasma phosphate	1.9 mmol/l
Plasma bilirubin	53 μmol/l
	contd

Plasma aspartate aminotransferase	32 543 IU/l
	(normal range 5–35)
Plasma alkaline phosphatase	178 IU/l
	(normal range 30–100)
Serum albumin	44 g/l
Hb	14.7 g/dl
Wbc	8.3×10^9/l
Platelets	210×10^9/l

What is the most likely diagnosis?

6.10

The following results were obtained from a healthy 57-year-old man at a routine medical examination:

Hb	19.2 g/dl
PCV	54%
RBC	6.6×10^9/l
MCV	83 fl
MCH	29 pg
MCHC	35 g/dl
Wbc	8.5×10^9/l
Platelets	200×10^9/l

Further investigations showed:

Red cell mass	normal
Arterial blood gases	
PaO_2	10.9 kPa
$PaCO_2$	4.2 kPa

(a) What is the most likely diagnosis?
(b) What treatment would you recommend?

Data Interpretation Paper 7

7.1

A 55-year-old man complains of chest pain. His blood pressure is 110/70 mmHg. His ECG on admission is shown.

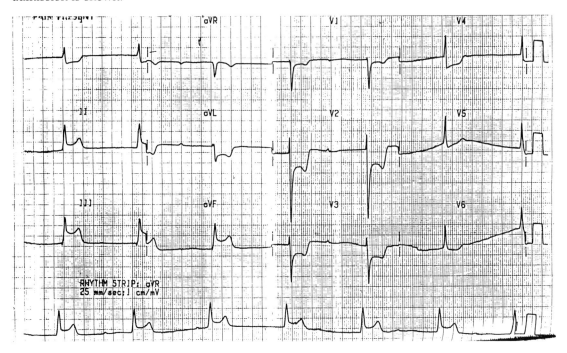

(a) What is the diagnosis?
(b) What is its anatomical basis?
(c) What treatment is indicated?
(d) Justify your treatment.

7.2

A 60-year-old woman is investigated for mild splenomegaly.
Investigations show:

Hb	8.7 g/dl
MCV	100 fl
Wbc	9.7×10^9/l
Platelets	187×10^9/l
Serum iron	44 μmol/l
	(normal range 13–32)
Serum ferritin	465 μg/l
	(normal range 15–300)
Blood film	normochromic and hypochromic erythrocytes

(a) What is the most likely diagnosis?
(b) How would you confirm this?

7.3

A 44-year-old clerk presents with anorexia and painless jaundice. On examination there is hepatosplenomegaly and a single axillary lymph node is palpated. He is sent home with a diagnosis of infectious hepatitis and seen in the out-patient department 2 weeks later. At this time he has a fever with ascites and ankle oedema.
Investigations show:

Hb	12.8 g/dl
Wbc	14.6×10^9/l
	neutrophils 85%
	lymphocytes 7%
	monocytes 5%
	eosinophils 1%
Serum albumin	23 g/l
Plasma bilirubin	125 mmol/l
Plasma alkaline phosphatase	380 IU/l
	(normal range 30–100)
Plasma alanine aminotransferase	38 IU/l
	(normal range 5–35)
Faecal fat	60 mmol/24 h
	(normal range 11–18 mmol/h)

(a) What is the likely diagnosis?
(b) Give three other possibilities.
(c) What investigation would you do to confirm the diagnosis?

7.4

A 65-year-old man with lymphoma who is being treated with cytotoxic drugs and steroids presents with polyuria. He also has a history of manic-depressive illness. After initial investigation, a water deprivation test was performed.

Date	Time	Urine osmolality (mOsm/kg)	Plasma osmolality (mOsm/kg)
25 August	1030	294	
	1130	243	
	1230	205	
	1300		289
	1330	203	
	1430	190	
	1600		299
	1630	250	
	1730	279	
	1730	DDAVP 2 mg given intramuscularly	
	1800	288	
	1830		289
	1830	276	
	1900	390	
	1930	411	
26 August	0030	486	
	0600	513	

(a) What initial investigation was performed before the water deprivation test?
(b) What is the cause of this patient's polyuria?
(c) What evidence is there that this has been an adequate test?

7.5

A 15-year-old Asian girl presents with increasing malaise and vomiting. She has recently emigrated to the UK.
   Investigations show:

Plasma sodium	127 mmol/l
Plasma potassium	4.7 mmol/l
Plasma urea	14 mmol/l
Plasma creatinine	135 μmol/l
Plasma bicarbonate	13 mmol/l
Plasma glucose	1.7 mmol/l

(a) What is the diagnosis?
(b) What important cause must you consider?

7.6

A 62-year-old man is referred to a renal physician for investigation of impaired renal function. He has lost 3 stone in weight over the previous 3 years, with intermittent episodes of nausea and vomiting.
   Investigations show:

Plasma sodium	134 mmol/l
Plasma potassium	3.0 mmol/l
Plasma bicarbonate	40 mmol/l
Plasma chloride	83 mmol/l
Plasma urea	15.4 mmol/l
Plasma creatinine	201 μmol/l
Plasma calcium	2.59 mmol/l
Plasma phosphate	1.06 mmol/l
Plasma alkaline phosphatase	69 IU/l *(normal range 30–100)*
Serum albumin	41 g/l
Abdominal ultrasound:	normal size kidneys; no evidence of obstruction; moderate enlargement of the prostate

(a) What is the diagnosis?
(b) How would you confirm this?

7.7

Following the death of his 39-year-old brother from a myocardial infarction, a 42-year-old man requests analysis of his serum lipids.
   Investigations show:

Plasma cholesterol	5.8 mmol/l *(normal range 4.7–6.2)*
Plasma HDL cholesterol	2.9 mmol/l *(normal range 0.96–2.0)*
Plasma LDL cholesterol	4.1 mmol/l *(normal range 2.4–5.0)*
Plasma triglycerides	8.1 mmol/l *(normal range 0.74–2.1)*

(a) What is the likely diagnosis?
(b) What single biochemical test would help confirm your diagnosis?

7.8

The MN blood group is determined by three genotypes, L^ML^M, L^ML^N and L^NL^N at the L locus. The distribution of genotypes in a population of 1000 individuals is:

Blood group	Genotype	Number of individuals
M	L^ML^M	450
MN	L^ML^N	500
N	L^NL^N	50

Assuming random mating between members of the population and no selective pressure, what will the genotype frequencies be in the next generation?

7.9

A 32-year-old renal transplant recipient attends a routine 3-month appointment at the transplant clinic. Since his last appointment, he has been well apart from several episodes of gout which have been managed by his general practitioner.
  Investigations show:

Plasma sodium	134 mmol/l
Plasma potassium	4.7 mmol/l
Plasma urea	14 mmol/l
Plasma creatinine	154 μmol/l
Plasma bicarbonate	23 mmol/l
Plasma urate	0.43 mmol/l
Hb	12 g/dl
Wbc	0.9×10^9/l

What is the likely cause of his low Wbc count?

7.10

A 10-year-old Greek boy presents with lethargy and reduced exercise tolerance. His mother says that he often complains of stomach pains.
  Investigations show:

Hb	9.8 g/dl
Wbc	7.8×10^9/l
MCV	65 fl
Platelets	430×10^9/l

(a) Give two likely diagnosis.
(b) Give four investigations which would clarify the problem.

Data Interpretation Paper 8

8.1

A 63-year-old man presents following an episode of loss of consciousness. His M-mode echo-cardiogram is shown.

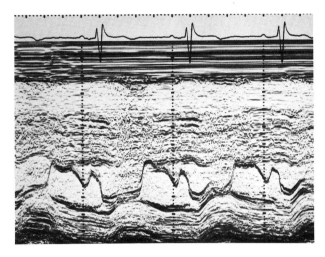

What is the diagnosis?

8.2

A woman who is in the 30th week of her second pregnancy is admitted because of ankle swelling and hypertension.
   Investigations show:

Plasma sodium	137 mmol/l
Plasma potassium	4.2 mmol/l
Plasma urea	11.7 mmol/l
Plasma creatinine	138 μmol/l
Hb	9.8 g/dl
Wbc	10.5×10^9/l
Platelets	40×10^9/l
Urinalysis	protein + + +
	blood + +
	glucose + + +
	contd

Investigations at antenatal clinic 18 weeks earlier:

Hb	12.6 g/dl
Wbc	10.7×10^9/l
Platelets	190×10^9/l
Blood glucose	4.5 mmol/l
VDRL	positive

(a) Suggest two possible diagnoses.
(b) Suggest three further investigations which would help establish the diagnosis.

8.3

This 69-year-old man complains of fluctuating tinnitus, vertigo and a feeling of fullness in his right ear. There is no air-bone gap.

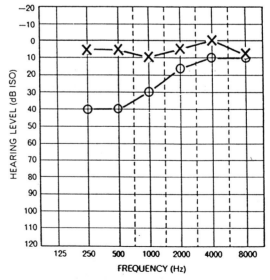

O – right
× – left

(a) What does this audiogram demonstrate?
(b) What is the likely diagnosis?

8.4

This is the ECG of a 45-year-old man who has been brought to casualty breathless.

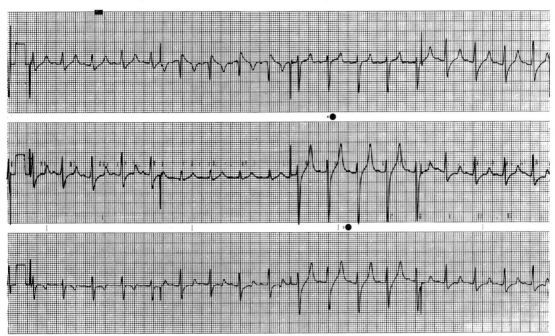

What is the cause of the ECG abnormalities?

8.5

A 21-year-old remains breathless after successful treatment of an apparently spontaneous pneumothorax. He mentions having to pass urine frequently. The chest X-ray report reads: 'Resolution of pneumothorax. Diffuse honeycomb appearance. Would be interested to know pathological diagnosis'.

Respiratory function tests show the following:

	Predicted	Actual
FEV_1 (l)	4.00	1.43
FVC (l)	4.93	2.93
FEV_1/FVC	48%	
TLC (l)	5.95	6.30
TL_{CO} (mmol/min/kPa)	10.64	5.1
K_{CO} (mmol/min(kPa/l)	1.90	1.4

(a) Describe two anatomical abnormalities and the findings in the respiratory function tests that support them.
(b) Suggest a diagnosis for the radiologist.

8.6

A 7-year-old boy presents with growth retardation.
Investigations were as follows:

Plasma sodium	142 mmol/l
Plasma potassium	4.2 mmol/l
Plasma urea	4.9 mmol/l
Plasma calcium	2.3 mmol/l
Plasma phosphate	0.3 mmol/l
Plasma alkaline phosphatase	175 IU/l *(normal range 30–100)*
Plasma glucose	4.3 mmol/l
Hb	12.9 g/dl
Wbc	9.2×10^9/l
Platelets	333×10^9/l
ESR	9 mm in the 1st hour

After 1 year of treatment with vitamin D he has grown 3 cm. Alkaline phosphatase is now 150 IU/l.

(a) What is the diagnosis?
(b) Suggest three radiological changes which you would expect to see.
(c) What investigation would confirm your diagnosis?
(d) Will his children need to see a doctor for the same problem?

8.7

Two blood samples taken from the same patient 10 min apart show the following results:

	First sample	Second sample
Hb	13.7 g/dl	14.4 g/dl
Wbc	7.4×10^9/l	8.0×10^9/l
Platelets	344×10^9/l	401×10^9/l
Plasma sodium	139 mmol/l	137 mmol/l
Plasma potassium	4.2 mmol/l	4.1 mmol/l
Plasma calcium	2.30 mmol/l	2.52 mmol/l
Serum albumin	42 g/l	47 g/l
Plasma glucose	4.3 mmol/l	4.5 mmol/l

What is the most likely explanation of the difference between the two sets of results?

8.8

A 35-year-old man complains of gradual weakness and increasing dyspnoea on exertion.
   Investigations show:

Plasma sodium	137 mmol/l
Plasma potassium	4.1 mmol/l
Plasma urea	5.7 mmol/l
Plasma creatinine	98 μmol/l
Plasma bilirubin	52 μmol/l
Plasma aspartate aminotransferase	21 IU/l *(normal range 5–35)*
Plasma alkaline phosphatase	75 IU/l *(normal range 30–100)*
Hb	9.1 g/dl
Wbc	2.1×10^9/l
Neutrophils	0.7×10^9/l
Platelets	50×10^9/l
MCV	98 fl
Reticulocytes	10%
Haptoglobins	negative
Hb electrophoresis	normal

(a) What is the likely diagnosis?
(b) What investigation would confirm this?

8.9

A 52-year-old man presents with recurrent transient ischaemic attacks which have persisted despite aspirin prophylaxis. The decision is made to anticoagulate him with warfarin. The following haematological results are obtained prior to his first dose.

Hb	13.8 g/dl
Wbc	8.9×10^9/l
Platelets	172×10^9/l
Prothrombin time	14 s *(control 12 s)*
Activated partial thromboplastin time	62 s *(control 35 s)*
Thrombin time	12 s *(control 12 s)*
Bleeding time	8 min *(control 5 min)*

(a) What is the diagnosis?
(b) What investigation would help confirm this?
(c) What is the cause of the prolonged bleeding time?

8.10

A 40-year-old woman is investigated as part of a routine life assurance medical.

Plasma sodium	135 mmol/l
Plasma potassium	4.1 mmol/l
Plasma urea	2.3 mmol/l
Plasma creatinine	45 μmol/l
Plasma bicarbonate	19 mmol/l
Plasma calcium	2.3 mmol/l
Plasma phosphate	1.4 mmol/l
Plasma glucose	6 mmol/l
Plasma bilirubin	7 μmol/l
Plasma aspartate aminotransferase	14 IU/l *(normal range 5–35)*
Plasma alkaline phosphatase	42 IU/l *(normal range 30–100)*
Serum albumin	34 g/l
Serum urate	0.12 mmol/l
Serum thyroxine	170 nmol/l *(normal range 70–140)*
Hb	9.8 g/dl
Wbc	5×10^9/l
Platelets	180×10^9/l
Urinalysis	glucose + +

What is the diagnosis?

Answers to Data Interpretation Paper 1

1.1

Accepted answers

(a) Atrial flutter with 2:1 atrio-ventricular block (100%)
    Atrial flutter (50%)

(b) Carotid sinus massage to increase the atrio-ventricular block (100%)

Explanation

In atrial flutter, the atrial rate is usually close to 300/min. Typically, 2:1 atrio-ventricular (AV) block results in a ventricular rate of 150. Thus whenever a patient has a ventricular rate of around 150, atrial flutter should be considered.

With a high degree of AV block, atrial flutter is easy to diagnose. The rapid atrial activity produces regular F waves. Often these appear as the characteristic 'saw tooth' baseline appearance. With 2:1 block, diagnosis can be more difficult, as alternate F waves can be superimposed on T waves. Temporarily increasing the degree of AV block should aid diagnosis; this could also be attempted pharmacologically, but as carotid sinus massage is simple, it is the best initial manoeuvre and attracts most marks. The figure below shows the ECG appearance after carotid sinus massage.

Note that 'atrial flutter with 2:1 block' attracts more marks than 'atrial flutter' alone.

> Remember to be as precise as possible in your answers. Don't allow yourself to give an incomplete answer.

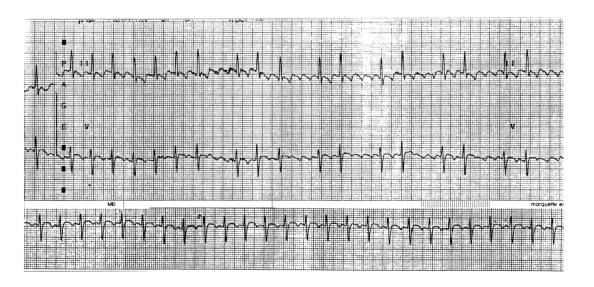

Interpreting ECGs

The ECG is one of the most important investigations to master for the data interpretation section, since examples are often included in papers. As it is one of the most common investigations performed in clinical practice, the examiners can reasonably expect candidates to interpret difficult examples. For this reason, a detailed approach to the ECG is given in Appendix B. This will allow you to pick up most abnormalities.

1.2

Accepted answers	*Rejected answers*
(a) Cushing's disease (100%) Pituitary-dependent Cushing's syndrome (100%)	Conn's syndrome Cushing's syndrome
(b) Excess glucocorticoid secretion Treatment of hypertension with diuretics	Excess aldosterone Secondary hyperaldosteronism
(c) Sampling of inferior petrosal sinuses for corticotrophin (100%) Magnetic resonance imaging of pituitary fossa (100%) CT reconstruction of pituitary fossa (100%) Chest X-ray (80%)	CT abdomen
(d) Transphenoidal microadenomectomy	Metyrapone Ketoconazole
(e) Transient cranial diabetes insipidus	

Explanation

Cushing's syndrome is defined by hypersecretion of cortisol. This can be demonstrated by a reliable 24-hour urine collection which contains more than 200 nmol of free cortisol or an elevated plasma cortisol level at 9 a.m. after administration of 1 mg of dexamethasone 9 h earlier. Having established cortisol hypersecretion, it is necessary to establish its cause.

Other types of Cushing's syndrome, such as hypothalamic-driven or the recently described adrenal hypersensitivity to gastrointestinal peptide, are rare.

Causes of Cushing's syndrome
- Cushing's disease
    Excess corticotrophin (ACTH) from a pituitary adenoma
- Ectopic source of ACTH
    Small cell carcinoma of the bronchus
    Small, undetectable carcinoid tumour
- Adenoma or carcinoma of the adrenal gland
- Corticosteroid or ACTH administration
- Alcohol excess

Diagnosis is classically sought on the basis of suppression by exogenous steroids.

Corticotrophin-driven Cushing's from a pituitary source will not be suppressed by low-dose dexamethasone (0.5 mg 6-hourly for 2 days) but will be suppressed by high doses (2 mg 6-hourly for 2 days). Ectopic corticotrophin-driven Cushing's and adrenal Cushing's will usually not suppress. However, these tests may be unreliable as 20% of pituitary-driven hypersecretion may not suppress, while benign ectopic sources may suppress.

Further refinement is possible by monitoring the corticotrophin response to intravenous ovine corticotrophin releasing hormone (CRH), providing the laboratory has a reliable corticotrophin assay. Cushing's disease is usually associated with an exaggerated rise in corticotrophin, while ectopic tumours do not respond. The most reliable method of detecting a pituitary source is to sample the inferior petrosal sinuses for corticotrophin and compare the ratio of the central to the peripheral level. Sensitivity is further increased by simultaneous infusion of the ovine releasing hormone.

The best way to image the pituitary fossa is by magnetic resonance imaging. Scanning the abdomen is useful if adrenal disease is suspected, and a chest X-ray may suggest an ectopic source.

The most likely diagnosis in this case is Cushing's disease, the usual cause of hypercorticolism in young women. The potassium is quite low for a patient with Cushing's disease, but the suppression of cortisol secretion with high dose dexamethasone is very suggestive of a pituitary source.

Definitive treatment for Cushing's disease is surgical. Medical therapy to control adrenal hypersecretion (metyrapone, ketoconazole or mifepristone) is used prior to surgery. Transient cranial diabetes insipidus is almost invariable for about 1 week post-operatively. No other complications are common.

Questions on Cushing's syndrome test your understanding of the pituitary adrenal axis. The questions are unlikely to be complicated provided the scheme outlined above is understood.

1.3

Accepted answer

Rhabdomyolysis

Explanation

The key to this question lies in the disproportionately raised creatinine compared with the urea level. An additional clue is the greatly raised phosphate and potassium. Renal failure resulting in a urea of only 22 mmol/l would not be severe enough to cause hyperkalaemia. Raised creatinine, phosphate and potassium levels are usually the result of muscle breakdown.

Diagnosis can be made by measurement of plasma creatine phosphokinase (CPK), which is usually markedly elevated.

Causes of raised creatine phosphokinase (CPK)
Muscle trauma
Rhabdomyolysis (bruises/contusion)
Intramuscular injections
Post DC shock
Myocardial infarction (note cardiac isoenzymes (CK-MB) can be distinguished from skeletal muscle isoenzymes)
Physical overexertion
Muscular dystrophy
Muscle inflammation
Polymyositis
Dermatomyositis

1.4

Accepted answer

1/150

The logic underlying this answer is as follows:
The probability of the patient being a heterozygous carrier is 2/3.
The probability that her fiancé has the abnormal gene is 1/25.
If both carry the gene, the probability of having a homozygous child is 1/4.
The overall chance of the patient having an affected child is thus:

$$2/3 \times 1/25 \times 1/4 = 1/150.$$

The difficult part of the question is working out the patient's chance of being a carrier. Cystic fibrosis has a recessive pattern of inheritance, thus the patient's parents must both be carriers. Hence, each of their children has a 1 in 4 chance of being homozygous and developing the disease, a 1 in 2 chance of being a heterozygous carrier, and a 1 in 4 chance of having two normal genes. However, because of her age, our patient knows she cannot by homozygous and that chance is removed. The probability that she is heterozygous then becomes 2 in 3.

This can be illustrated by a simple analogy. If a bag contains one black ball (representing the homozygous state), two red balls (the heterozygous state), and one white ball (normal), the chance of picking a red ball is 1 in 2. If the black ball is then removed, corresponding to our patient knowing she cannot be homozygous, the chance of picking a red ball becomes 2 in 3.

Note that you are given no information about the health of the fiance's family, but it is reasonable to assume there is no history of cystic fibrosis and that he has a 1 in 25 chance of carrying the gene.

> This is a difficult question, not least because it has more to do with mathematics than medicine. When you encounter a difficult question, miss it out so that you can return to it once you have finished the rest of the questions. There is nothing worse than spending a long time on an impossible question only to find that you have left yourself too little time to do the remaining, easier questions.

1.5

Accepted answers

(a) Restrictive defect

(b) Asbestos related pleural thickening
(100%)

Mesothelioma (50%)

Rejected answers

Obstructive lung defect

Pulmonary fibrosis
Emphysema

Explanation

Respiratory (or pulmonary or lung) function tests are a favourite examination question. Usually, the relative change in FEV_1 and FVC (often expressed as FEV_1/FVC) will allow you to determine whether you are dealing with a predominantly restrictive or obstructive defect. In an obstructive defect, FEV_1 falls more than FVC and the ratio FEV_1/FVC decreases. In a restrictive defect, both fall and the ratio may be normal or increased.

In a patient with a restrictive defect, the next important question is whether the defect arises from pulmonary fibrosis (or oedema, which produces the same picture), or from abnormalities of the rib cage (used here to include the pleura, chest wall and respiratory muscles). To answer this, it is important to have an understanding of TL_{CO} and K_{CO}, as determined by carbon monoxide gas transfer.

A patient inhales a mixture of air, helium and carbon monoxide, holds his breath for 10 s and exhales. Helium is inert, so its dilution in a sample of exhaled air allows the **volume of distribution** of the gas mixture to be calculated. Carbon monoxide diffuses rapidly across alveolar walls, so its dilution in the exhaled mixture depends on the volume of blood in contact with the alveolar volume, which in turn is a function of the nature of the alveolar walls, capillary volume and the pattern of ventilation and perfusion in the lungs. The carbon monoxide gas transfer for the whole or total lung (TL_{CO}) is expressed as the uptake of the gas per unit partial pressure gradient of carbon monoxide (mmol/min/kPa). When this is corrected for the volume of distribution, the transfer coefficient, K_{CO} (mmol/min/kPa/l), is obtained.

Pointers to pulmonary fibrosis are a reduced TL_{CO}, reduced transfer factor (K_{CO}) or low PaO_2 with normal or low $PaCO_2$. These changes are a manifestation of the thickening of alveolar walls and obliteration of alveolar capillaries by pulmonary fibrosis.

In extensive pleural disease, relatively small alveolar volumes are created by a rigid,

constrictive pleural cage. However, alveolar walls are normal, allowing unimpaired gas transfer at the level of the single alveolus. As a result, single breath carbon monoxide transfer (i.e. for the whole lung) is reduced, but when this is divided by the reduced value for alveolar volume to obtain the K_{CO}, a raised value is obtained.

Causes of a raised K_{CO} include
Pulmonary haemorrhage
Polycythaemia
Left-to-right shunts
Bronchial asthma
Pneumonectomy
Neuromuscular weakness
Skeletal deformity

In this question, FVC is reduced much more than FEV_1, suggesting a restrictive defect. The restriction may arise from pulmonary fibrosis or from extrapulmonary disease such as pleural thickening. The raised K_{CO} suggests extrapulmonary disease with unimpaired gas transfer. The hint of asbestos-related disease may lead you to suggest mesothelioma as an underlying diagnosis, but although this tumour may present with this clinical picture due to pleural thickening, a pleural effusion is common. Mesothelioma may thus gain some marks but is less precise in the absence of more characteristic evidence. Other diseases of the chest wall might also gain some marks, but the possibility of asbestos exposure in the occupational history is too strong for the examiners to ignore!

1.6

Accepted answers

Ventricular septal defect with a left-to-right shunt (100%)

Ventricular septal defect (50%)

Explanation

In the normal heart oxygen saturations in the right chambers and vessels should be uniformly lower than those on the left side. Abnormal saturations imply the presence of an abnormal communication between the two sides of the heart. When asked to interpret abnormal saturations, you should comment on two things – the level of communication and the direction of the shunt.

If a right-sided chamber or vessel has a saturation higher than expected, this implies blood has reached it through a shunt from the left. Similarly, a left-sided chamber or vessel with a lower saturation than expected implies a shunt from the right. The anatomical level of the shunt can be determined by looking at the saturations in anatomical order. All right-sided measurements (SVC, IVC, RA, RV, and PA) should be more or less the same as each other, as should all left-sided measurements (LA, LV, and aorta). The first chamber to deviate from this rule is the site of the 'step-up' or 'step-down'.

In this question a step-up clearly occurs at the level of the right ventricle. This implies a left-to-right shunt at the level of the ventricles

(a VSD) because well-oxygenated blood from the left ventricle has mixed with venous blood in the right ventricle. The step-up occurs as blood cannot flow from right ventricle to right atrium across the tricuspid valve. A step-down at the level of the left ventricle would also imply a VSD, but with a right-to-left shunt.

Cardiac catheterization data frequently appear in the examination, but only a limited number of conditions are likely to come up. It is sensible to concentrate on these, which include:

- Atrial septal defect
- Ventricular septal defect
- Patent ductus arteriosus
- Pulmonary stenosis
- Aortic stenosis
- Mitral stenosis

Combinations of abnormalities may also come up, e.g. Fallot's tetralogy.

1.7

Accepted answers

(a) Wilson's disease

Rejected answers

Fanconi syndrome
Other causes of type 2 renal tubular acidosis (e.g. cystinosis, heavy metal poisoning)

(b) Serum caeruloplasmin level (100%)
Liver biopsy (100%)

Urinary copper excretion (80%)
Slit lamp examination (80%)

Analysis of urine for aminoaciduria
Ammonium chloride loading test

(c) Kayser–Fleischer rings
Hepatomegaly
Spasticity
Parkinsonism
Muscle wasting
Chorea
Dysarthria
Dysphagia

Explanation

The combination of these observations should suggest Wilson's disease. This is a good Membership question because its multisystem features allow the same information to be presented in numerous ways. It is an auto-somal recessive disorder characterized by an inability to excrete copper. It most commonly presents in the second or third decade, at which stage Kayser–Fleischer rings are invariably present, but the diagnosis cannot be excluded without slit-lamp examination. Any movement disorder may be present, including chorea, parkinsonism, spasticity or cerebellar ataxia. Patients with neurological disease invariably have liver disease which may have been 'silent'. However, liver disease may dominate the picture with acute hepatic failure, chronic active hepatitis and cirrhosis. Presentations involving other systems occur more rarely (except in MRCP papers!), but may be renal as in this case, with proximal renal tubular acidosis, renal glycosuria and bi-carbonate wasting, or endocrine (e.g. amenor-rhoea). Overall frequencies of the initial pre-dominant presentation are hepatic (42%), neurological (34%), psychiatric (10%), renal (1%), or haematological/endocrinological secondary to hepatic dysfunction (12%).

Diagnosis requires the presence of low serum caeruloplasmin levels and Kayser–Fleischer rings, or excess copper in liver biopsy; in practice the implications of the diagnosis are so great that patients are usually subjected to biopsy. Other cholestatic dis-orders (e.g. primary biliary cirrhosis) also cause excess hepatic copper deposition, but not to such a degree and usually in the face of increased caeruloplasmin.

Treatment is lifelong administration of penicillamine; hypersensitivity can usually be controlled by prednisolone. Withdrawal of penicillamine may be fatal. Patients with fulminant hepatic failure or progressive liver disease despite treatment may be considered for transplantation.

1.8

Accepted answers

(a) Visceral leishmaniasis (100%)
Brucellosis (100%)
Tuberculosis (100%)

Lymphoma (50%)

(b) Bone marrow biopsy (or aspirate) and culture (100%)
Liver biopsy and culture (100%)
Blood culture (100%)

Splenic aspirate (50%)

Rejected answers

Mantoux test
Montenegro test

Explanation

The answer to this question should centre on causes of hepatospenomegaly, as discussed in Case Histories question 8.1.

Although other diagnoses are possible, the nationality of the patient should immediately suggest visceral leishmaniasis. The investiga-tions support this diagnosis.

Kala-azar or visceral leishmaniasis is caused by *L. donovani*. It is transmitted by the bite of a sandfly. The organisms multiply within the macrophages in the reticuloendothelial system and the amastigotes are often seen on liver or bone marrow biopsies or in splenic aspirates. The clinical picture is chronic and non-specific, with intermittent fever, weight loss, lethargy, wasting, epistaxis, cough and diarrhoea, amongst other symptoms. A normocytic normochromic anaemia, neutropenia, thrombocytopenia, hypoalbuminaemia, hypergammaglobulinaemia, massive splenomegaly, lymphadenopathy, and hepatomegaly can occur. In HIV-positive patients, the illness is more cryptic and the clinical features are atypical.

Diagnosis is made by demonstrating the Leishman–Donovan bodies. Pentavalent antimony (sodium stibogluconate) or pentamidine can be used in treatment.

> In questions such as this, remember **the diagnosis can often be based on the differential diagnosis of a single clinical sign**, in this case hepatospenomegaly.

1.9

Accepted answers

(a) Lead encephalopathy (100%)

   Subacute sclerosing panencephalitis (SSPE) (50%)

(b) Examination of blood film for basophilic stippling (100%)

   Electroencephalogram (50%)
   Blood lead level (50%)
   Urinary porphyrins (50%)

Explanation

Questions on CSF are common and easy to answer. It is important to have a list of causes of each of the common abnormalities. There are relatively few causes of a raised CSF protein with a normal cell count, as in this case.

> **Causes of a raised CSF protein with a normal cell count**
> Guillain–Barré syndrome (and some other peripheral neuropathies, unlikely to feature in examinations)
> Spinal block
> Lead encephalopathy
> Subacute sclerosing panencephalitis

In this question, the raised CSF pressure suggests lead encephalopathy, the preferred answer which would attract most marks. The additional clue is the reference to the working class family, perhaps unfairly suggesting a house with lead plumbing. In SSPE, the EEG is characteristic and the diagnosis can be confirmed by an oligoclonal band in the CSF which cross-reacts with the measles antigen.

> When the examiners request a *simple* examination they are asking for a test which the laboratory can perform quickly and cheaply, and which supports the diagnosis but does not necessarily confirm it. Thus blood lead levels or CSF electrophoresis for oligoclonal band might confirm the diagnosis, but would take a long time to do so; thus they would attract fewer marks as an answer to this question.

1.10

Accepted answers

(a) There is no significant difference between the mean arterial pressures of the control and treated groups after 3 months of treatment.

(b) Normal distribution
Gaussian distribution

(c) 1/100
1%

Explanation

You would be unlucky to encounter a statistics question, but statistics do turn up reasonably often in the viva in part II so it could equally occur in the written paper. However, if you read the chapter summaries of an O level book in statistics (which will take about 20 min), you will know 90% of the statistics you need for your medical career, never mind the MRCP examination!

Student's *t* test is one of the most commonly used statistical tests in clinical studies. It is a parametric test, which means it is only valid if applied to data that is normally distributed.

Significance is usually arbitrarily defined as a *p* value of less than 0.05, which means that there is less than a 1:20 (5%) probability that the difference between two groups is due to chance alone.

Answers to Data Interpretation Paper 2

2.1

Accepted answer

True posterior myocardial infarction (100%)

Myocardial infarction (25%)

Explanation

The R-waves and depressed ST segments in the anterior leads represent the changes of acute infarction in the posterior wall viewed, as it were, from behind, and hence reversed. The physiological Q waves sometimes seen in V_1 in a normal ECG are lost. Dominant R waves in V_1 might suggest right ventricular hypertrophy, but there is no right axis deviation, and the T waves in the left ventricular leads are upright.

> **Causes of a dominant R wave in V_1**
> Posterior myocardial infarction
> Right bundle branch block
> Wolff–Parkinson–White type A
> Right venticular hypertrophy
> Mirror image dextrocadia

2.2

Accepted answer

Mitral stenosis

Explanation

There are five modes of echocardiography in general use: M-mode, two-dimensional (2-D), pulsed Doppler, continuous wave Doppler and colour flow mapping. In the MRCP examination it is probable that you will only be asked to interpret M-mode or 2-D echocardiograms.

M-mode echocardiograms are obtained using a fixed unidirectional beam which records the movement of anatomical structures lying in a line immediately below the transducer. The direction of the beam is first chosen from the two-dimensional scan. There are three common M-mode recordings: a view of the aortic valve at the level of the aortic root and left atrium; a transverse view across the left ventricular cavity at the level of the tips of the mitral leaflets; and a view across the left ventricular cavity just below the mitral valve

tips. Of these, it is the last which is usually shown in the MRCP, illustrated in a normal subject in the figure overleaf. The following normal structures are identified:

A. Interventricular septum
B. Left ventricular cavity
C. Anterior leaflet of the mitral valve
D. Posterior leaflet of the mitral valve
E. Posterior left ventricular wall
F. Potential pericardial space

> Echocardiography is a specialized investigation. Few candidates will have been asked to interpret echocardiograms prior to Membership. In specialized, more difficult techniques such as this, it is probable that you will only encounter a few conditions. These should be predicted and remembered prior to the examination.

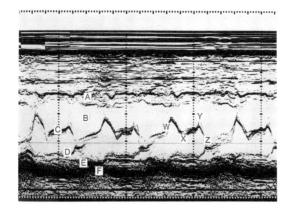

These are the echocardiograms you are most likely to encounter in the examination:
Mitral stenosis
Hypertrophic cardiomyopathy
Pericardial effusion
Left atrial myxoma
Aortic incompetence

Adopt a standard approach to looking at the echocardiogram. First, examine the potential pericardial space; if there is an echo-poor area here, then there is a pericardial effusion. Second, look at the interventricular septum – is this hypertrophied compared to the posterior wall? If so, consider a diagnosis of hypertrophic cardiomyopathy, in which case you will often also see anterior movement of the mitral valve during systole (i.e. upwards on a conventionally reproduced echocardiogram), the so-called 'systolic anterior movement' or 'SAM'.

Finally, examine the mitral valve and its pattern of movement. The normal mitral valve opens fully (W), then moves back to a semi-closed position (X) during mid-diastole; it opens further during atrial systole (Y) and then closes at the onset of ventricular systole (Z). If it is thickened, and its normal M-shaped movement during diastole becomes a straight line, then the diagnosis is mitral stenosis (compare the figure here with the echocardiogram shown in the question. Rather than showing the characteristic M-shaped movement [WXYZ in the figure here] the anterior leaflet of the mitral valve adopts the box-like shape of the M-mode echo in the question). Flutter on the valve during diastole (this looks like a high-frequency saw tooth movement) indicates the regurgitant stream of blood from the aortic root and hence aortic incompetence.

In left atrial myxoma, the mitral 'box' will be filled with echos as the valve orifice is occupied by the tumour.

2.3

Accepted answers

(a) Chronic lymphocytic leukaemia

(b) Haemolytic anaemia
Reticulocytosis
Alcohol abuse
Megaloblastic anaemia
Folate deficiency
Vitamin B_{12} deficiency

Explanation

Chronic lymphocytic leukaemia is the most common leukaemia in the West, and its incidence increases with age. The important features for the Membership examination are that it is usually a B cell leukaemia, where the prognosis depends on tumour bulk, as is reflected in the staging. Where disease load is small (e.g. few nodes involved, Hb greater than 10 g/dl, platelets greater than 100×10^9/l) the prognosis is no worse than that of matched controls. The important complications are autoimmune haemolytic anaemia (5% of patients have positive direct antiglobulin tests) and infections, as the patients have depressed humoral and cell mediated immunity.

It is worth remembering the causes of macrocytosis – they are relatively few, and the abnormality is likely to occur in Membership questions.

In this case the elevated MCV is most likely due to a reticulocytosis (as reticulocytes are larger than erythrocytes the automated cell counter reads the average cell size as increased), alcohol consumption (which causes macrocytosis through its effects on lipid metabolism and hence the erythrocyte membrane) and megaloblastic anaemia due to poor diet.

Causes of macrocytosis
Megaloblastic anaemia
Reticulocytosis
Alcohol
Liver disease
Hypothyroidism
Myelodysplasia
Less common causes in the Membership examination:
Multiple myeloma (due to associated B_{12} and folate deficiency and haemolysis)
Acquired sideroblastic anaemia
Aplastic anaemia
Drugs, e.g. azathioprine, phenytoin

2.4

Accepted answers	*Rejected answers*

(a) Familial Mediterranean fever (or relapsing polyserositis) with amyloid-related malabsorption and nephrotic syndrome

Amyloidosis or FMF alone
Chronic pancreatitis
Lymphoma
Coeliac disease

(b) Rectal biopsy (100%)
Jejeunal biopsy (100%)

Amyloid scan
Skin biopsy
Jejeunal aspiration

(c) Colchicine

(d) Hypoalbuminaemia

Pleurisy

Explanation

Familial Mediterranean fever (FMF) or relapsing polyserositis is an autosomal recessive disease particularly common in non-Ashkenazi Jewish, Turkish, Armenian and Middle Eastern Arab populations. It is characterized by recurrent serositis presenting with fever, abdominal pain, pleurisy and arthritis, with resolution between attacks. Amyloidosis is a complication, often leading to renal failure, which can be prevented by prophylaxis with colchicine. The molecular basis of the disorder is unknown, although recent reports suggest that the gene responsible maps to the short arm of chromosome 16.

This man has two causes for his hypoalbuminaemia: he has nephrotic syndrome and malabsorption, both due to amyloid deposition.

Malabsorption in Membership
Malabsorption may be defined as a disturbance in the transfer of nutrients from the intestinal lumen into the circulation. Note that this covers a wider spectrum of disease than steatorrhoea. It is important to be able to distinguish the mechanisms of malabsorption on the basis of diagnostic tests which you should know for the examination.

General tests:
These are fairly routine tests which would suggest malabsorption, e.g. macrocytic anaemia associated with low red cell folate and, later, low serum B_{12}, low serum albumin, calcium and potassium.

Three day stool fat excretion:
This should be performed whilst the patient is on a defined fat diet (100 g/day). The documentation of steatorrhoea suggests (a) intraluminal hydrolysis due to lack of lipase activity (e.g. pancreatic disease, Zollinger–Ellison syndrome); (b) fat solubilization due to bile salt deficiency (e.g. biliary obstruction, interrupted enterohepatic circulation, bacterial overgrowth); (c) decreased reabsorption due to resection of small bowel, damage to mucosal cells or increased transit; or (d) impaired transport of chylomicrons. In other words, it is a rather non-specific investigation (which most labs hate doing!).

Jejeunal or duodenal biopsy:
This allows examination of the mucosa for characteristic lesions (Whipple's disease, amyloidosis, lymphoma) or for pathogens (e.g. *Giardia*, *Cryptosporidia*). Serial biopsies may be necessary to document a response to therapy as diagnostic (coeliac disease). The procedure also allows jejeunal aspiration for the diagnosis of bacterial overgrowth.

D-Xylose excretion:
Failure to absorb xylose and excrete it in the urine is an indicator of loss of absorptive surface in the gut. A normal test may suggest pancreatic rather than jejunal disease, but there is a high false-negative rate. In addition D-xylose excretion is abnormal in renal disease, hypothyroidism, ascites, after gastric surgery, with diarrhoea (which may be provoked by the xylose!) and in the elderly, as well as in malabsorptive states. In short, many gastroenterologists find it of limited value.

Bile acid breath test:
In bacterial overgrowth, deconjugation of bile acids occurs early in the small intestine, rather than in the large bowel. Hence if a test dose of $[^{14}C]$-glycocholic acid is given by mouth, the $^{14}CO_2$ level in expired air is high and peaks early when there is bacterial overgrowth. Measuring the amount of hydrogen in expired air following a dose of lactulose works on a similar principle. If transit time is fast, the breath test will give false positives.

Schilling test:
Where absorption (and hence urinary excretion) of $[^{57}Co]$-cyanocobalamin is impaired, its failure to significantly improve when given with intrinsic factor suggests malabsorption due to ileal desease. However, it also occurs in bacterial overgrowth and pancreatic disease. In the latter case this is due to the requirement for pancreatic proteolysis to release B_{12} for binding to intrinsic factor.

Tests of pancreatic exocrine function:
Endoscopic retrograde cholangiopancreatography (ERCP) allows visualization of the pancreatic duct, biopsy and aspiration of duodenal contents following stimulation with secretin and/or cholecystokinin.

Para-amino benzoic acid (PABA)/bentiromide test: $[^{14}C]$-PABA conjugate is ingested and ^{14}C measured in the urine over a 6-h period. This conjugate is hydrolysed by pancreatic chymotrypsin.

Pancreolauryl (fluorescein dilaurate) test: this is a substrate for pancreatic aryl esterase, releasing the fluorescein which can then be measured in the urine.

As we have discussed, all these tests have significant problems and several in combination are often needed to make a diagnosis.

2.5

Accepted answers

(a) Pulmonary embolism

(b) Severe asthma
   Pulmonary oedema
   Pneumothorax
   Pulmonary haemorrhage

Rejected answers

Opiate overdose
Brain stem stroke
Emphysema
Chronic airways limitation

Explanation

A useful way to interpret arterial blood gases in respiratory disease is to first distinguish acute from chronic hypoxaemia, and then consider the presence or absence of carbon dioxide retention.

- Marked acute hypoxaemia without CO_2 retention is characteristic of pulmonary embolism, asthma, pulmonary oedema, pulmonary haemorrhage and pneumothorax.
- Acute hypoxaemia with CO_2 retention implies a failure of ventilation rather than a problem at the site of gas exchange. Thus there may be failure of the respiratory drive (e.g. respiratory depressants), failure to transmit this drive (e.g. Guillain-Barré, syndrome, myasthenia gravis) or mechanical problems of lung expansion (e.g. chest wall injury, severe obstructive defect, stiff lungs due to severe oedema).
- Chronic hypoxaemia without CO_2 retention can develop as a result of any chronic lung disease where ventilation is relatively unimpaired: pulmonary fibrosis, chronic airflow limitation and emphysema and recurrent thromboembolism.
- Chronic hypoxaemia with CO_2 retention will develop as the end-stage of chronic hypoxaemia without CO_2 retention, or when a combination of the above develops.

The acute onset and occupational history are typical clues to suggest pulmonary embolism as a cause of hypoxaemia. The non-invasive investigation to confirm this is a ventilation-perfusion isotope scan (not the shorthand VQ scan). Unfortunately, this may not provide a definitive diagnosis and if the clinical suspicion is high, pulmonary angiography may be indicated. This is the gold standard of diagnosis. (For a discussion on the pros and cons of VQ scans versus pulmonary angiography, see the *British Medical Journal* 1992; **304**: 1126–7.)

Massive pulmonary embolism is defined as obstruction of 50% or more of the pulmonary arterial bed on angiography. In the real world investigations take time and may not be available in the same hospital. Initiation of therapy may be necessary without definitive diagnosis. If there is systemic hypotension, hypoxia, and evidence of shock in the appropriate clinical context, thrombolytic therapy is warranted; if this is contraindicated, pulmonary embolectomy is the only viable option.

Smaller pulmonary emboli may cause infarction with or without pleuric chest pain, with recurrent episodes giving rise to a syndrome of sustained pulmonary hypertension.

> The difficulty in this type of question is not the initial answer (the likely diagnosis) but in obtaining full marks for all the other possible diagnoses requested in the next part of the question.

2.6

Accepted answer

(a) Renal failure secondary to multiple myeloma

(b) Serum electrophoresis for paraprotein (100%)
    Radiological skeletal survey (100%)
    Bone marrow aspiration (100%)
    X-ray of affected site (lumbar spine) (100%)
    Examination of peripheral blood film (100%)

    Urine electrophoresis for Bence Jones protein (10%)

Explanation

This question provides a good example of basing a differential diagnosis on a combination of key abnormalities. The constellation of abnormalities to consider here are: renal failure, hypercalcaemia and elevated serum protein. Base the diagnosis on the causes of hypercalcaemia.

Causes of hypercalcaemia
Primary hyperparathyroidism
Tertiary hyperparathyroidism
Malignancy with ectopic hormone production
Myeloma
Sarcoidosis
Thyrotoxicosis
Milk–alkali syndrome
Vitamin D overdosage
Artefactual (venous stasis during collection)

The only cause that will produce a raised total protein of this degree **and** renal failure is myeloma. The history fits this diagnosis.

Note that renal failure usually presents with hypocalcaemia, not hypercalcaemia; tertiary hyperparathyroidism will cause a raised calcium, but only after long-standing renal failure (the patient here has probably developed renal failure over a course of months); sarcoidosis can occasionally cause renal failure and raised γ-globulins.

Finally, the reason the answer 'urine electrophoresis for Bence-Jones protein' attracts so few marks is because the patient is anuric! Admittedly, you might be able to obtain some residual urine following catheterization, but the point is that you should make sure that you aren't giving silly answers. Always read the question carefully to avoid this.

2.7

Accepted answer

Blood specimen analysed after standing overnight

Rejected answer

Haemolysed sample

No patient well enough to remain an out-patient could have these blood results. There must be shum mistake shurely doctor! There is evidence of cell lysis from the high potassium and phosphate (normally intracellular). However, the low glucose implies continued metabolism (which is prevented by collecting it in a fluoride tube). These observations make it unlikely that this is merely a haemolysed sample. In fact, this specimen was analysed only after being left unattended for a whole weekend.

2.8

Accepted answer

(a) Primary biliary cirrhosis

(b) Anti-mitochondrial antibodies
    Liver biopsy

Explanation

Primary biliary cirrhosis (PBC) characteristically occurs in middle-aged women. Itching is a common feature and is caused by retention of bile salts. Anti-mitochondrial antibodies directed against the inner casing of mitochondria are found in 90% of patients. Liver biopsy usually shows piecemeal necrosis, prominent septa and infiltration with lymphocytes and plasma cells. Inflammation and resulting fibrosis around the bile ductules result in cholestasis with consequent pruritus, hypercholesterolaemia, and malabsorption of fat.

2.9

Accepted answers

(a) Axonal peripheral neuropathy

(b) Hereditary sensorimotor neuropathy type 2 (100%)
    Vitamin B$_{12}$ deficiency (100%)

    Charcot–Marie–Tooth disease (50%)

Rejected answers

Demyelinating peripheral neuropathy
Peripheral neuropathy

Hereditary sensorimotor neuropathy type 1

Explanation

The approach to this question involves the classification of neuropathies into demyelinating and axonal. Demyelinating neuropathies cause a marked reduction in nerve conduction velocity, commonly measured at the median and/or common peroneal nerves, as well as a reduction in action potentials. In axonal neuropathies, conduction velocities are well preserved.

There is sufficient data here for you to lose marks for failing to specify an axonal neuro-pathy. Charcot–Marie–Tooth disease, an obsolete term for HSMN-1 and -2, would gain some marks.

Important causes of axonal neuropathy include HSMN-2, diabetes, B$_{12}$ and folate deficiency, renal failure, carcinomatous neuropathy and most drug-related neuropathies (e.g. vincristine, isoniazid).

Important demyelinating neuropathies include HSMN-1, diabetes, Guillan–Barré syndrome and the 'acquired demyelinating neuropathies'.

2.10

Accepted answers

(a) Dermatomyositis

(b) Malignancy (100%)
    Neoplasia (100%)

Explanation

Insidious symmetrical proximal muscle weakness results from muscle inflammation in dermatomyositis. The disease mainly affects women of between 40 and 50 years.

Dysphagia, dysphonia, respiratory weakness, cardiomyopathy, lung collapse and fibrosis may develop. Approximately 25% of patients have a purple skin rash especially in areas exposed to sunlight, and some may have a 'heliotrope' (a lilac blue flower) rash around the eyes. Telangiectasia may be found on the face, arms and chest. Diagnosis is by muscle enzymes (CPK and serum aldolase), electromyogram and muscle biopsy.

Malignancy is present in approximately 10% of all patients and in over 50% of men presenting over the age of 50 years. The most commonly associated tumours are carcinoma of the lung, prostate, ovary, breast, uterus or large intestine. Treatment or removal of the tumour may result in a remarkable improvement in the muscle disease.

Causes of a raised CPK are given in the answer to Data Interpretation question 1.3.

Answers to Data Interpretation Paper 3

3.1

Accepted answers	*Rejected answer*

(a) Atrial septal defect with left to right shunt (100%)

  Pulmonary stenosis (100%)

  Pressure gradient between right ventricle and pulmonary artery (or across pulmonary valve) (100%)

  Atrial septal defect (50%)

  High systolic pressure in right ventricle (or RV hypertension) (50%)

  Step-up in oxygen saturation from vena cavae to right atrium (50%)

  Increased O_2 on right side (25%)

  Left to right shunt (25%)

(b) Turner's syndrome

  Post-rubella infection

Rejected answer

Right ventricular hypertrophy

Explanation

A guide to the interpretation of cardiac catheterization data is given in the answer to Data Interpretation question 1.6.

3.2

Accepted answers

(a) J wave

  Atrial fibrillation

  Prolonged Q-T interval

  Muscle tremor (shivering) artefact

(b) Hypothermia

Explanation

The point behind this question is to remind you of (a) 'ECG syndromes' and (b) the 'non-cardiac' causes of ECG abnormalities – metabolic and drug effects. If you are having difficulty interpreting an ECG it is always worth running through a list of these. Below is a list of those you may meet in the exam and what you should be looking for.

Causes of 'non-cardiac' ECG abnormalities

Calcium effect
Hypercalcaemia
　　Shortened Q-T interval

Hypocalcaemia
　　Prolonged Q-T interval

Potassium effect
Hyperkalaemia
　　Peaked, tall T wave
　　Widened QRS complex
　　Diminution of P wave amplitude
　　Diminution of R wave amplitude

Hypokalaemia
　　Flattened or inverted T wave
　　Prominent U wave
　　Depressed S-T segment
　　Prolonged P-R interval

Digitalis effects
Downward sloping S-T segment depression (reversed tick), particularly in leads V5 and V6
Shortened Q-T interval
Sinus bradycardia
1st degree A-V block
2nd degree A-V block
Atrial and nodal tachycardias

Hypothermia
　　J wave
　　Sinus bradycardia
　　Atrial fibrillation
　　Ventricular fibrillation
　　Muscle tremor (shivering) artefact
　　Prolonged Q-T interval

3.3

Accepted answers

(a) Autosomal dominant

(b) 1:2

Explanation

The family pedigree shows the characteristic features of autosomal dominant inheritance in which a monogeneic disorder is passed on to offspring by one parent and the disease manifests itself clinically in the heterozygous state. Approximately 1/2 of offspring are affected, irrespective of whether they are male or female. Each generation is affected.

The probability of an affected offspring from the consanguinious marriage shown in the pedigree is still 1/2. In this disease consanguinity is irrelevant, because we already know that one parent does not carry the abnormal gene and the other is heterozygous. The question is designed to fool you.

3.4

Accepted answers	Rejected answers
(a) Type 1 (distal) renal tubular acidosis	Type 2 (proximal) renal tubular acidosis Osteomalacia
(b) Renal calculi Nephrocalcinosis Looser's zones	
(c) Osteomalacia	Hypocalaemia

Explanation

In renal tubular acidosis (RTA) there is a failure to acidify urine to a level appropriate for blood pH; systemic acidosis is therefore not corrected. Unlike renal failure, anions such as sulphate and phosphate are filtered normally and are therefore unavailable to balance the loss of bicarbonate; electrical neutrality is instead maintained by renal chloride absorption resulting in a **hyperchloraemic metabolic acidosis with a normal anion gap**.

In proximal (Type 2) renal tubular acidosis, there is a diminished renal bicarbonate threshold because bicarbonate reabsorption in the proximal tubules is incomplete. The increased urinary bicarbonate excretion lowers the plasma bicarbonate concentration until a new steady state is reached. At this stage the urine is free of bicarbonate and has an acid pH to match the systemic acidosis. Proximal RTA in its primary form usually presents in infants with failure to thrive, polyuria and growth retardation. Secondary forms may occur in patients with generalized proximal tubular damage due to cystinosis, Wilson's disease or myeloma, and after renal transplantation. There is no metabolic bone disease and nephrocalcinosis is unusual.

The pathophysiology of distal (Type 1) RTA is complex, but can be thought of in simple terms as a failure of hydrogen ion secretion in the distal tubules. The urine is therefore never acid, even in the presence of systemic acidosis.

The systemic acidosis reduces tubular re-absorption of calcium, resulting in hyper-calcuria and secondary hyperparathyroidism: nephrocalcinosis and bone disease are therefore characteristic. Distal RTA is most commonly a dominantly inherited condition.

In both disorders acidosis provokes potassium loss and hypokalaemia, and patients often complain of weakness as a result.

The diagnosis of distal RTA can be made in a patient with a hyperchloraemic metabolic acidosis and a urinary pH above 5.5. If acidosis is mild or absent, an ammonium chloride loading test may be necessary. Normal individuals should lower their urinary pH to below 5.5; patients with distal RTA will not.

Proximal tubular acidosis should be considered especially in patients with hyperchloraemic acidosis and associated features such as glycosuria and aminoaciduria. If the metabolic acidosis is severe enough, an early morning urine of pH 5.5 or less supports the diagnosis. If a low urinary pH is not found, an ammonium chloride test should be performed to exclude the diagnosis of distal RTA. A definitive diagnosis can be made by bicarbonate titration. The characteristic finding is an elevated urinary excretion of bicarbonate in the face of a normal plasma bicarbonate.

This patient has distal RTA as the urine pH is high despite systemic acidosis, and because there is clinical evidence of bone disease and nephrocalcinosis.

3.5

Accepted answer

Repeat blood gas analysis

Explanation

The low bicarbonate and high carbon dioxide should generate a repiratory acidosis. In view of the pH, there must be an error.

Such questions are unlikely, but they do provide a test of your understanding by showing that you can recognize inconsistencies. Do not be shy of exposing these, having excluded all other possibilities.

A second trick to watch for is an initial investigation which is inappropriate. For example, in this question a case could be made for giving peak expiratory flow rate as the answer, since in real life this would almost certainly be performed before blood gas analysis. However, repeating the blood gases is a better answer as it shows that you have spotted an error, the results of which need to be explained.

3.6

Accepted answers	*Rejected answers*
(a) The microscopic appearance of the blood film	White cell differential count Mean corpuscular volume
(b) Microangiopathic haemolytic anaemia (MAHA) Disseminated intravascular coagulation (DIC)	Anaemia secondary to PV haemorrhage Septic bone marrow failure
(c) Septic abortion Retained products of conception	Pre-eclampsia Amniotic fluid embolus

Explanation

Microangiopathic haemolytic anaemia (MAHA) and disseminated intravascular coagulation (DIC) are two popular conditions which often come up in the Membership. They may present similarly, i.e. bleeding and with similar aetiologies.

In MAHA, damage to small vessel vascular endothelium causes adherence of fibrin fragments which trap and fragment erythrocytes and platelets. In pure MAHA clotting is therefore normal. The blood film is characteristic, with red cell fragments and fibrin strands, and nucleated red cells due to the reticulocytosis.

DIC results when a variety of insults cause simultaneous thrombosis and fibrinolysis within the circulation. This may be low-grade and compensated and therefore clinically inapparent, or may be unbalanced with consumption of clotting factors and haemorrhage. In pure DIC, any anaemia is due to bleeding and clotting is deranged due to consumption of coagulation factors. FDPs are elevated as fibrinolysis is also occurring. The trauma to red cells from deposits of fibrin in small vessels may itself be sufficient to cause a MAHA.

The common causes of both these disorders are a variety of obstetric disasters, sepsis and carcinoma. Less common causes of MAHA which may occur in Membership type questions are:

- Haemolytic uraemic syndrome and thrombocytopenic purpura
- Accelerated hypertension
- Scleroderma crisis
- Drugs: oral contraceptive, cyclosporin A, mitomycin

In the case presented here, a white cell differential count will not contribute to the diagnosis. Similarly, various indicators of haemolysis (e.g. elevated methaemalbumin, unconjugated bilirubin, reduced haptoglobins) will not establish the type of haemolysis. The mean corpuscular volume could theoretically help to distinguish anaemia due to bleeding from that due to haemolysis. However, the anaemia is too acute to be reflected by a real fall in MCV, and this parameter may be elevated by the reticulocytosis. The presence of leucocytosis argues against a diagnosis of bone marrow failure secondary to sepsis. Finally, whilst pre-eclampsia and amniotic fluid embolus are causes of MAHA in pregnancy, they are diseases of the second and third trimesters.

3.7

Accepted answers

Churg–Strauss syndrome (100%)

Polyarteritis nodosa (50%)

Rejected answer

Wegener's granulomatosis

Explanation

This patient clearly has a systemic disease, and you are being called on to recognize a syndrome. The biggest clue is the positive anti-neutrophil cytoplasmic antibody (ANCA), which suggests an autoimmune disease, particularly a vasculitis. The non-vasculitic causes of a positive ANCA generally give a perinuclear staining pattern, p-ANCA (as here), but anti-myeloperoxidase antibodies are not present. ANCA, particularly p-ANCA, is currently only used as diagnostic corroboration. A more detailed discussion of ANCA is to be found in Case History question 3.3.

The purpuric skin lesion represents a cutaneous vasculitis. The history of nasal involvement, eosinophilia and the lack of any renal impairment or an active urinary sediment suggests either Churg–Strauss syndrome or classical polyarteritis nodosa (PAN); the history of asthma makes the former much more likely.

3.8

Accepted answers   *Rejected answers*

(a) Tuberculous meningitis

(b) Staining of CSF for AAFB (Ziehl–   Culture of CSF for AAFB
     Neelson or immunofluorescent stain-   Culture of sputum for AAFB
     ing) (100%)   Mantoux test
     Chest X-ray (100%)

     Microscopic examination of urine
     (50%)
     Ziehl–Neelson staining of sputum
     (50%)

Explanation

The differential diagnosis must centre around   The history is most suggestive of tuber-
causes of lymphocytosis in the CSF.   culous meningitis. Investigations should be
                                                 aimed at confirming this as quickly as possible.

Causes of lymphocytosis in the cerebrospinal fluid	
Tuberculous meningitis	Cerebral abscess
Viral meningitis	Cerebral toxoplasmosis
Fungal meningitis	Sarcoidosis
Meningovascular syphilis	CNS lymphoma/leukaemia

3.9

Accepted answers

(a) Chronic active hepatitis

(b) Wilson's disease (100%)
     Drugs (e.g. methyldopa) (100%)
     Hepatitis C or E (100%)
     α-1-Antitrypsin deficiency (100%)
     Autoimmune (100%)

Explanation

The differential diagnosis can be based upon   Patients with primary biliary cirrhosis are
the liver function tests, which show hepato-   older and the jaundice is cholestatic.
cellular jaundice.

Causes of hepatocellular jaundice

Infections	Toxins
Viral	Drugs
Hepatitis A, B, C, D, E	Nitrofurantoin
EBV	Halothane
CMV	Isoniazid
HIV	Inherited disorders
Arboviruses	Wilson's disease
Spirochaetes	Galactosaemia
Leptospira	Autoimmune disease/connective tissue
Protozoa	disorders
Toxoplasma	SLE
Amoeba	Scleroderma

3.10

Accepted answers

(a) Systemic lupus erythematosus (SLE)

(b) Anti-double stranded DNA antibodies (anti-dS DNA antibodies)

(c) Depression
Psychosis
Seizures
Cranial nerve lesions
Cerebellar ataxia
Meningitis
Transverse myelitis
Encephalopathy
Cerebrovascular accidents
Transient ischaemic attacks

Explanation

Clinical features of SLE include the following manifestations in the approximate frequency shown in brackets: musculoskeletal (95%), cutaneous (80%), fever (77%), splenomegaly (70%), CNS (60%), renal (50%), pulmonary (50%), cardiovascular (40%) and normocytic normochromic anaemia (25%).

Nearly 80% of patients with SLE have antinuclear antibodies. Anti-double stranded DNA antibodies are more specific in diagnosis. Forty per cent of patients with SLE have rheumatoid factor and about 10% give a false positive VDRL test. Complement levels are usually decreased in active SLE.

Answers to Data Interpretation Paper 4

4.1

Accepted answers

Left atrial myxoma (100%)

Atrial myxoma (75%)

Rejected answers

Left atrial ball thrombus
Infected vegetation

Explanation

This echocardiogram shows the classic picture of a left atrial myxoma. The tumour mass can be seen at the mitral orifice during diastole. A ball thrombus almost never prolapses like this.

Note that left atrial myxoma is likely to attract more marks than simply atrial myxoma.

A guide for the interpretation of M-mode echocardiograms in Membership is given in the answer to Data Interpretation question 2.2

4.2

Accepted answers

(a) Gilbert's syndrome

(b) No treatment is required

Explanation

Inherited in an autosomal dominant mode, Gilbert's syndrome (disease) is a common congenital hyperbilirubinaemia found in 2–5% of the population. Fasting, stress, intercurrent illness and intravenous nicotinic acid produce a rise in plasma bilirubin and icterus may be noticeable.

The prognosis of this condition without treatment is excellent.

4.3

Accepted answers

(a) Anaemia of chronic disease secondary to chronic renal failure
    Thalassaemia trait

(b) Haemoglobin electrophoresis

Explanation

This is a difficult question in which all but two of the data are abnormal. There is a clearly discernible pattern of results which, taken with the history, suggests chronic renal failure. However, this alone cannot explain the grossly depressed MCV of 58 fl. The logical approach is to consider the differential diagnosis of a microcytic anaemia.

Causes of microcytic anaemia
Iron deficiency
Anaemia of chronic disease
Thalassaemia
Sideroblastic anaemia
Aluminium toxicity

The most common cause of a microcytic anaemia is iron deficiency. This diagnosis can be confirmed by a low serum iron, low serum ferritin and a high total iron binding capacity (TIBC) or transferrin. The reticulocyte count is appropriately low for the degree of anaemia.

The anaemia of chronic disease is usually normocytic or **mildly** microcytic. Both serum iron and TIBC are low and ferritin normal or raised.

In thalassaemia traits, the MCV is always very low for the degree of anaemia, which is often mild or absent. Serum iron and ferritin are normal.

Sideroblastic anaemias are characterized by ring sideroblasts in the bone marrow. The disorder may be congenital or acquired: the MCV is often very low in the former but often raised in the latter. Serum iron and ferritin are both raised.

The anaemia of aluminium toxicity is seen exclusively in patients with long-standing dialysis-dependent renal failure who have either used dialysates containing high levels of aluminium or who have received large amounts of aluminium-containing phosphate binders.

The patient in this question has chronic renal failure and a severe microcytic anaemia. The anaemia of chronic disease (associated in this case with renal failure) undoubtedly contributes to her anaemia, but does not explain the low MCV. The normal ferritin makes iron deficiency and congenital sideroblastic anaemia unlikely. The history suggests that the patient has not yet received renal replacement therapy (i.e. dialysis), so aluminium toxicity is unlikely. Thalassaemia trait could be clinically silent and still cause this degree of microcytosis. This should be confirmed by haemoglobin electrophoresis.

This is another situation where marks are earned by providing the most complete answer. The answer to (a) should be 'anaemia of chronic disease due to chronic renal failure'. To omit either part is to provide an inferior answer.

4.4

Accepted answers

(a) Anti-glomerular basement membrane disease
   Goodpasture's disease

(b) Anti-GBM antibody titre
   Renal biposy

(c) Vasculitis
   Systemic lupus erythematosus

Explanation

This question concerns the differential diagnosis of 'pulmonary-renal syndromes', i.e. disorders which affect both kidneys and lungs. This has already been discussed in Case History 3.3.

In this case you are forced to make a single choice for a diagnosis. The history is typical for anti-glomerular basement membrane disease, and as this is the best-known acute disease to affect both lungs and kidneys, the College would expect it as an answer.

4.5

Accepted answers

(a) Paget's disease of bone (osteitis deformans)

(b) X-ray of affected site
      Bone scan

(c) Biphosphonates
      Simple analgesia

Explanation

The differential is that of a very high alkaline phosphatase with a normal calcium in an elderly gentleman. The likely diagnosis is Paget's disease of bone. Rarely it may be confused with osteomalacia, but the calcium is usually low in this condition.

The causes of an elevated alkaline phosphatase are discussed in the answer to Case Histories Section 1 answer 8.2.

4.6

Accepted answers

(a) Tri-iodothyronine thyrotoxicosis

(b) Free tri-iodothyronine (T3)

(c) Radioiodine

Rejected answers

Facticious hyperthyroidism due to self-medication with thyroxine.
Non-compliance with medication

Increase carbimazole dose
Propanolol

Explanation

The examiners like to test your understanding of thyroid function tests by giving results in situations where they can be misleading. These include:

- T3 thyrotoxicosis, as here. Replapse of hyperthyroidism while on carbimazole may be due to T3 thyrotoxicosis.
- Subclinical thyroid disease. TSH is elevated but T4 is within the normal range. Currently accepted practice is to treat these patients with thyroxine to suppress TSH into the normal range.
- Pregnancy. Thyroxine-binding globulin levels (TBG) increase during pregnancy so total thyroxine levels rise. TSH is still a reliable indicator of thyroid status, except in the first trimester, where it is often suppressed due to the thyrotrophic action of human chorionic gonadotrophin.
- Coincident disease. In acute illness, TSH is often suppressed, probably through several mechanisms. In chronic illness, the tests are often difficult to interpret; in chronic renal failure thyroid hormone levels are often diminished but TSH maintained.
- The oral contraceptive stimulates TBG production in much the same way as pregnancy. Iodine-containing drugs, such as amiodarone, can inhibit thyroid hormone secretion, leading to a rise in TSH. Corticosteroids and dopaminergic drugs cause suppression of TSH secretion.

The important overall message is that TSH is a reliable indicator of thyroid status except when the hypothalamic-pituitary axis is manipulated, as in pregnancy, dopamine agonists, etc.

The diagnosis in this question must be T3 thyrotoxicosis as either of the other possibilities would cause a rise in T4.

Relapse of thyrotoxicosis while on carbimazole is a relative indication for definitive treatment (radioiodine or thyroidectomy). It is now more usual to treat women of child-bearing age with radioiodine, as there is no evidence of any risk from gonadal irradiation providing pregnancy is avoided for the following 4 months.

It is useful to remember a list of causes of hyperthyroidism:

The following account for over 90% of cases:

Graves' disease
Toxic multinodular goitre
Toxic solitary nodule

The 'common' rare causes that may crop up are:

TSH-driven hyperthyroidism
Factitious hyperthyroidism
Exogenous iodide (Jod–Basedow phenomenon) e.g. drugs, X-ray contrast materials
Thyroiditis
McCune–Albright syndrome, as one of many possible endocrinopathies

---

4.7

Accepted answers

(a) Lyme disease (100%)

Sarcoidosis (50%)
Systemic lupus erythematosus (50%)

(b) Serum IgM antibodies specific for *Borrelia burgdorferi* (100%)

Kveim test (50%)
Serum angiotensin converting enzyme levels (50%)
Liver biopsy (50%)
Titre of serum antibodies to double stranded DNA (50%)

Explanation

The differential diagnosis is that of a raised CSF protein and a lymphocytosis. This is much wider than that of a raised CSF protein alone. The examiners are therefore keen on this type of question, and will expect you to use all the clues they provide to make a definitive diagnosis. In this case, the clues suggest Lyme disease as the likely diagnosis; you should expect fewer marks for other diagnoses.

Causes of raised CSF protein and CSF lymphocytosis

Infection

   Lyme disease – diagnostic clues include rash, cranial nerve palsy, low CSF glucose

   Tuberculous meningitis – usually occurs in immigrants or immunosuppressed (AIDS); patients often have hydrocephalus with ataxia, drowsiness, high CSF pressure and low glucose

   Fungal meningitis – usually immunosuppressed patients with low CSF glucose

   Syphilis – may be asymptomatic, presenting only with positive serum syphilis serology

   Viral meningitis – no focal neurological signs, normal CSF glucose and often normal protein

   Viral encephalitis – presents with abnormal behaviour often with convulsions; normal CSF glucose but raised protein

Non-infectious

   Sarcoidosis – usually some other clue such as a skin rash. (Glucose only slightly reduced)

   Multiple sclerosis – usually a classical clinical presentation (e.g. optic neuritis). CSF shows a slight lymphocytosis (less than 50 cells/mm^3) normal glucose and only moderately elevated protein

   Leptomeningeal secondary neoplasms

   Others, such as systemic lupus erythematosus and Beçhet's disease, are very unusual

---

4.8

Accepted answer

(a) Respiratory alkalosis

(b) Hysterical overbreathing

(c) Reassurance and rebreathing into a bag

Explanation

The differential diagnosis is that of a respiratory alkalosis.

The likely diagnosis in this case is hysterical hyperventilation. Reassurance and rebreathing into a bag is all that is required. Sedation should be used with caution in extreme cases.

Remember that hyperventilation can also occur as a result of a metabolic acidosis.

Causes of respiratory alkalosis

Hysterical overbreathing

Continuous pain

Stimulation of respiratory centre by hypoxia

   Pulmonary oedema

   Pneumonia

   Pulmonary collapse or fibrosis

   Pulmonary embolism

Excessive artificial ventilation

Brain stem lesions

Salicylate poisoning

Acute liver failure

Hyperventilation due to metabolic acidosis

Diabetic ketoacidosis

Salicylate overdose

Lactic acidosis

Renal failure

Renal tubular acidosis

Transplantation of ureters into colon

Drugs, e.g. acetazolamide

4.9

Accepted answers

(a) Impaired auditory acuity in right ear at
4 kHz (4000 Hz), both by bone and air
conduction (100%)
Sensorineural hearing loss in the right ear
at 4 kHz (4000 Hz) (100%)

(b) Noise-induced hearing loss following shotgun use

Explanation

Audiograms will be unfamiliar to many candidates, so it is probable they will be fairly easy to interpret. There will be a maximum of four lines plotted on the graph, representing air conduction and bone conduction for each ear. You are less likely to be shown cases of conductive deafness (air conduction lost compared to bone conduction) than sensori-neural loss (air and bone conduction both lost), since the former are more in the domain of the ENT surgeon than the physician.

The general format of an audiogram is to place increasing sound frequency on the horizontal axis. The vertical axis shows hearing level in decibels, decreasing towards the top of the axis (in fact, to be accurate, the vertical axis really represents hearing level compared to a representative control group against which the audiometer has been calibrated). In other words, the higher the plot, the better the hearing, as the patient is detecting a given frequency at a lower hearing level.

You will often be asked to describe an audiogram. Remember to specify which ear(s) are/is affected and the relative effect on air and bone conduction. In this question, you have been told that there is no air-bone gap, i.e. bone conduction is no greater than air con-duction. As this would not be the case if the

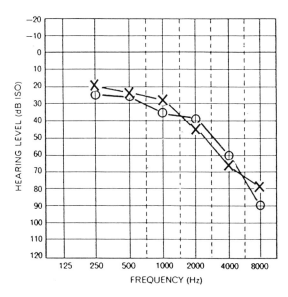

O – right
X – left

question illustrated a conductive hearing loss, the defect here is sensorineural.

> Do not be afraid to include in your answer facts that you have been given in the question. In this question, although you have already been told that there is no air-bone gap, you should still include the word 'sensorineural' in the answer. You are telling the examiner that you know when something is important.

Deterioration in auditory acuity with age is normal. It is usually symmetrical and affects high tone acuity more severely. An example is illustrated in this figure. Asymmetrical high tone sensorineural deafness suggests a cerebellopontine angle lesion such as acoustic neuroma or meningioma. Low tone fluctuating sensorineural hearing loss is suggestive of Ménière's disease.

Noise-induced sensorineural hearing loss secondary to the use of a shotgun only affects the contralateral ear, as the ipsilateral ear is protected by the butt of the gun. The game-keeper in this case is left handed, so his right ear has been affected by the noise of the gun. In contrast, an explosion next to an individual will affect the ipsilateral ear more. Industrial noise injury is often bilateral, resulting in symmetrical 4 kHz dips.

4.10

Accepted answers

(a) Benign paraproteinaemia
     (benign monoclonal gammopathy)

(b) Bone marrow aspiration

(c) Regular follow-up in clinic

Rejected answers

Myeloma

Chemotherapy

Explanation

Benign paraproteinaemia can be defined as the presence of a monoclonal protein without evidence of malignant disease. Up to 1% of the population may have benign monoclonal proteins, the incidence increasing with age. Most are of the IgG class, but IgM and IgA paraproteins also occur. Diagnostically, the difficulty is in differentiating paraproteinaemia in an asymptomatic individual from early myeloma.

Between 10 and 20% of benign paraprotein-aemias develop into myelomas, but this may not be apparent for several years. Thus regular follow up is recommended.

Finally, some benign monoclonal proteins are the result of strong antigenic stimulus, such as persistent parasitic infection.

The following features help distinguish benign from malignant paraproteinaemias:
- The paraprotein concentration is less than 20 g/dl
- There is no immune paresis, i.e. other immunoglobulin classes are not suppressed
- There are no free light chains (Bence–Jones protein) in the urine
- The bone marrow contains less than 15% plasma cells
- There are no radiological bone lesions
- There is no increase in paraproteinaemia with time

Answers to Data Interpretation Paper 5

5.1

Accepted answers

(a) First degree heart block
ST segment depression in leads V3, V4, V5, V6, I and aVF
Left atrial hypertrophy
Prominent U waves

(b) Hypokalaemia

Explanation

Another illustration of 'non-cardiac' causes of ECG abnormalities, discussed in the answer to Data Interpretation question 3.2. The main ECG manifestations of a low serum potassium are flattening or inversion of the T waves, depression of the ST segment, prolongation of the PR interval and prominent U waves. The relative loss of the T wave, and the loss of the P wave in the U wave as the PR interval is prolonged, may result in a U wave being mistaken for a T wave. Other non-specific manifestations of hypokalaemia include an increased frequency of ventricular extrasystoles and enhanced digoxin toxicity.

5.2

Accepted answers

Right ventricular infarction (100%)

Right heart failure following a myocardial infarction (50%)

Explanation

This question makes two important points.

> Firstly, the answer to data questions may be in the clinical presentation, and it is important to extract as much information as possible from the history provided.

Thus the predominance of signs of right ventricular impairment with no response to diuretics suggests that the right ventricle has infarcted.

Secondly, cardiac pressure questions are easy to answer, even without knowledge of normal values. Basic physiology tells you that left-sided filling pressures should be higher than right-sided; here the end-diastolic or filling pressure of the right ventricle is higher than the end diastolic pressure in the left ventricle, which is reflected by the left atrial and hence pulmonary wedge pressures.

Right ventricular infarction is usually associated with inferior infarction. The principle differential diagnosis is pulmonary embolism (different presentation, elevated pulmonary artery pressures). The answer 'right heart failure following a myocardial infarction' is less precise and might attract fewer marks.

5.3

Accepted answer

1 : 32

Explanation

The answer is best explained using the following pedigree:

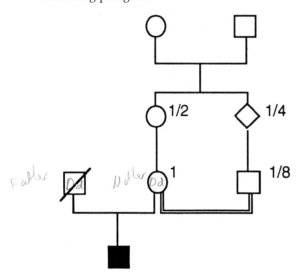

Figures show probability that an individual is heterozygous for an abnormal gene.

In order to have an affected child with an autosomal recessive disease, the mother must be a carrier, i.e. heterozygous. If her cousin is also heterozygous, the probability of them having an affected child is $\frac{1}{2} \times \frac{1}{2} = \frac{1}{4}$. As shown in the pedigree, the probability that her cousin is also heterozygous for the abnormal gene is $\frac{1}{8}$. Thus the overall probability that a child will be affected is $\frac{1}{2} \times (\frac{1}{2} \times \frac{1}{8}) = \frac{1}{32}$.

5.4

Accepted answers

(a) Dermatitis herpetiformis

(b) Coeliac disease

(c) Jejunal biopsy

Explanation

The investigations are consistent with malabsorption and the rash suggestive of dermatitis herpetiformis (DH). DH is associated with coeliac disease (CD) and responds to treatment with dapsone or a gluten free diet. Both DH and CD have a strong association with HLA-B8 and HLA-DR3.

Apart from nutritional deficiencies, complications of coeliac disease include:
    Development of malignancy
        Increased risk of all GI malignancies
        T cell lymphoma of small bowel
    Myopathy
    Neuropathy
    Splenic atrophy

Other common causes of small bowel malabsorption are:
    Bacterial overgrowth
    Crohn's disease
    Lymphoma
    Parasites
        Giardia
        Capillaria
        Strongyloides
    Partial gastrectomy
    Jejunal diverticulosis

A general guide to the investigation of malabsorption is given in the answer to Data Interpretation question 2.4.

Causes of itching
- Primary skin conditions
    Eczema
    Scabies
    Lichen planus
    Drug
        Reactions
        Side-effects (e.g. chloroquine)
    Viral exanthems (e.g. chickenpox)
    Tinea
    Onchocerciasis
    Larva migrans
    Urticaria
- Systemic conditions
    Liver disease
    Chronic renal failure
    Lymphoma
    Polycythaemia
    Pregnancy
    Iron deficiency

5.5

Accepted answers

(a) Felty's syndrome

(b) Splenomegaly

Explanation

Felty's syndrome is defined as the association between rheumatoid arthritis, splenomegaly and leucopenia. Thrombocytopenia may also occur, as in this case. Other features include anaemia, skin ulceration and weight loss. Typically, Felty's syndrome is found in patients with severe rheumatoid arthritis. Its pathogenesis is unclear, but splenomegaly is probably the major factor contributing to the neutropenia. The main risk is recurrent infection. Treatment is indicated if it causes recurrent infection, persistent skin ulceration, thrombocytopenic bleeding or severe anaemia. The response to steroid therapy is inconsistent. Splenectomy will increase the white cell count and reduce the risk of infection.

Many candidates will be familiar with this syndrome and we would expect them to get the correct answer without difficulty. We include the case because syndromes such as this make nice Membership questions, and are worth remembering.

Causes of neutropenia	Cyclical
Part of general pancytopenia	Inherited
Bone marrow failure	Viral infections
Splenomegaly (e.g. Felty's syndrome)	Severe bacterial infection
Paroxysmal nocturnal haemoglobinuria	Autoimmune neutropenia
(but reticulocytosis often present)	SLE
Drug-induced	Hypersensitivity and anaphylaxis

5.6

Accepted answers	*Rejected answers*
(a) Hypothyroidism	Polymyositis or dermatomyositis, muscular dystrophy
(b) Dry skin (100%) Thin hair (100%) Bradycardia (100%) Delayed relaxation of tendon reflexes (100%) Myotonia (100%)	
(c) (Highly sensitive) thyroid stimulating hormone (TSH) assay Thyroxine assay Thyroid antibodies	Electromyography Muscle biopsy

Explanation

This patient has a number of classical features of hypothyroidism, none of which usually dominates the presentation and all of which occur in other disorders. However, it is difficult to think of another condition which includes a myopathy with only mildly elevated muscle enzymes, hyponatraemia and a macrocytic anaemia.

Hyponatraemia in hypothyroidism is due to inappropiate secretion of antidiuretic hormone. The macrocytosis is probably related to increased lipid deposition in the red cell membrane. The muscle enzymes are insufficiently raised for there to be significant myositis.

When discussing thyroid function tests, it is worth specifying highly sensitive TSH assays, as the older assays are not capable of distinguishing between low normal values and the suppressed levels of hyperthyroidism.

The thyroid antibodies usually measured are anti-microsomal and anti-thyroglobulin antibodies. Both are present in signficant titre in Hashimoto's thyroiditis. A more likely aetiology in a woman of this age is spontaneous atrophic non-goitrous hypothyroidism. This is also an organ-specific autoimmune disease with lymphoid infiltration of the thyroid and TSH receptor blocking antibodies (cf. receptor stimulating antibodies in Graves' disease). These antibodies are not useful clinically.

Treatment of primary hypothyroidism is aimed at keeping the TSH within the normal range in conjunction with clinical findings.

> **The aetiology of primary hypothyroidism can be classified as follows:**
> Non-goitrous
>   Spontaneous atrophic
> Goitrous
>   Hashimoto's thyroiditis
>   Drug-induced (lithium, amiodarone)
>   Iodine deficiency
>   Dyshormonogenesis (e.g. Pendred's syndrome)
>   Post-ablative (postoperative or radioiodine – often transient if develops within 6 months of therapy)

5.7

Accepted answer

(a) Haemolytic–uraemic syndrome

(b) Fragmented erythrocytes
    Spherocytes

Explanation

The haemolytic–uraemic syndrome typically occurs in children shortly after a febrile illness associated with diarrhoea. HUS causes a microangiopathic haemolytic anaemia, as discussed in the answer to Data Interpretation question 3.6. In this case, the combination of the history, low platelet count and anaemia should provide sufficient evidence for the diagnosis to be made. Do not let the age of the patient fool you – the condition can also occur in adults.

5.8

Accepted answers

(a) Reversible airway obstruction with raised K_{CO} (100%)

    Reversible obstructive defect (50%)

(b) Atopic asthma (100%)

    Occupational asthma (50%)

Rejected answers

Obstructive defect

Farmer's lung

Explanation

The respiratory function tests show the characteristic features of the obstructive defect of asthma: an obstructive defect with a raised K_{CO}. In addition they show reversibility – defined as an improvement of 15% or greater in FEV_1 after bronchodilators.

> Be particularly careful to provide very full answers if the question seems easy.

The second question can be rephrased as this: could it be anything other than asthma? The occupational history is compatible with a diagnosis of farmer's lung, a form of extrinsic allergic alveolitis. However, even acute EAA with wheeziness is usually associated with a restrictive defect on respiratory function testing. In addition, the reversibility of the airways obstruction argues against EAA where reversibility of any obstruction present may be attenuated because of the predominance of inflammation over bronchospasm. The overall respiratory picture is more in keeping with atopic asthma which may indeed present only with a dry cough. The history of hay fever confirms his atopy.

> The examiners are testing your self-confidence as well as your knowledge. Neither is much use without the other. Learn to stick by your guns.

5.9

Accepted answers

(a) Partially treated bacterial meningitis (100%)
    Cerebral abscess (100%)
    Fungal meningitis (100%)
    Diabetes mellitus (100%)

    Tuberculous meningitis (25%)

(b) Acid/alcohol-fast stain for mycobacteria
    Indian-ink stain for fungi
    Countercurrent immunoelectrophoresis for
        bacterial antigens (remains positive even
        when culture is negative)

Explanation

Tuberculous meningitis is a less good diagnosis because of the relatively low proportion of lymphocytes in the CSF, and (of much less help to us) the information that there is no growth on culture, which might have included culture for mycobacteria. (Although we do not know for how long it is cultured, one may reasonably conclude that the question assumes the cultures are negative after 2–3 days only.)

Ambiguous results may suggest interference by doctors, and should alert you to partially treated conditions or their recovery phase. Similarly, relatively unusual conditions may produce unusual CSF pictures, such as fungal meningitis.

Always be aware of the probably irrelevant information which may provide the last answer for which you are struggling – in this case the elevated blood glucose level.

> If an apparently irrelevant piece of information is abnormal, think again – it may not be irrelevant.

5.10

Accepted answers

Renal artery stenosis (100%)
Reno-vascular disease (100%)

Rejected answers

Conn's syndrome
Primary hyperaldosteronism
Cushing's syndrome
Adrenal adenoma

Explanation

Potassium is a crucial investigation in the initial assessment of secondary hypertension.

Causes of hypokalaemia and hypertension
- Diuretics
- Primary hyperaldosteronism (Conn's syndrome)
    Adrenal adenoma
    Adrenal hyperplasia
    Adrenal carcinoma
- Secondary hyperaldosteronism
    Renal artery stenosis
    Cirrhosis
    Nephrotic syndrome
    Renin-secreting juxtaglomerular tumour
- Mineralocorticoid effect of excess gluco-corticoids
    Cushing's disease and syndrome
    Steroid therapy

Conn's syndrome

Questions about Conn's syndrome usually carry some hint towards the diagnosis other than hypokalaemia, e.g. nocturia or the typical biochemical picture of a hypokalaemic alkalosis and serum sodium of more than 140 mmol/l. The basis of most tests for Conn's syndrome is to demonstrate (a) hypokalaemic alkalosis, (b) increased plasma aldosterone in circumstances where aldosterone secretion would normally be suppressed and (c) low plasma renin activity. Suppression of aldosterone secretion can be attempted by lying the patient down,

infusing saline, administering a high salt diet or giving fludrocortisone. Aldosterone can be measured in plasma or urine. Plasma renin activity will fail to rise during volume depletion (e.g. standing up) if it is suppressed by autonomous aldosterone secretion. Many antihypertensive drugs may interfere with these tests. If antihypertensive medication cannot be stopped, nifedipine is probably the least disruptive agent.

Secondary hyperaldosteronism

The common stimulus in the various forms of secondary hyperaldosteronism appears to be reduced renal perfusion, due to renal artery stenosis or intravascular depletion. This results in the clinical syndrome of hypertension, oedema, low serum potassium and raised renin. The usual cause of renal artery stenosis in an elderly population is atheroma at the origin of the artery from the abdominal aorta. Occasionally the artery will be involved in an abdominal aortic aneurysm.

In this question the examiners are trying to get you to answer Conn's syndrome. However, there are pointers towards renal artery stenosis:

- there is oedema and the serum sodium is less than 140 mmol/l; both suggest secondary hyperaldosteronism
- there is evidence of generalized atheroma.

The mild renal failure does not help differentiate since hypertension of any cause may result in renal impairment.

Answers to Data Interpretation Paper 6

6.1

Accepted answers

(a) Gram-negative septic shock (100%)

Septic shock (75%)

(b) Metabolic acidosis (100%)

Rejected answer

Hypotension

Explanation

The combination of systemic hypotension, low left and low right heart pressures means either hypovolaemia or septic shock (or a combination of both, which is often the case in clinical practice). In this case, the key to the correct diagnosis is the cardiac output (or cardiac index, which is the cardiac output/m^2 of body surface area). When this increases and the blood pressure falls, as here, then systemic vascular resistance must have fallen (as cardiac output = blood pressure/systemic vascular resistance). This is the predominant situation during the vasodilatation of septicaemic shock. In hypovolaemia, systemic vascular resistance should rise as a result of vasoconstriction.

Note, however, that septic shock and hypovolaemia often occur together and that the immediate management of septic shock usually involves fluid replacement.

Septic shock leads to a metabolic acidosis because of poor tissue perfusion. The respiratory centre will respond with hyperventilation in order to lower blood PaCO$_2$.

6.2

Accepted answers

(a) X-linked dominant
Autosomal dominant

(b) 1:2

Explanation

The great majority of X-linked disorders are recessive, but a few are dominant. The following criteria apply to all X-linked disorders:

- Male-to-male transmission never occurs as a father cannot pass on his X chromosome to his son.
- All daughters of an affected male will receive the abnormal gene. If the disease is X-linked recessive they will be carriers; if the disease is X-linked dominant they will all be affected.

- Unaffected males never transmit the disease to sons or daughters.
- If X-linked recessive, half the sons of female carriers will be affected; similarly if X-linked dominant, half the sons of affected females will be affected.
- Half the daughters of carrier females will be carriers; in X-linked dominant disease, half the daughters of affected females will be affected.

This family tree may superficially resemble a pattern of autosomal dominant inheritance. However, closer inspection reveals that the disease is never transmitted from father to son, characteristic of X-linked inheritance. Furthermore, all the daughters of affected males are also affected, indicating X-linked dominant inheritance.

On the basis of a pedigree alone, it is difficult to distinguish between the two modes of inheritance. Although the presence of male-to-male inheritance in a pedigree excludes X-linked inheritance, the converse is not true. X-linked dominant disorders are rare enough for you to be wary of claiming this mode of inheritance even if no cases of male-to-male inheritance are seen in a large pedigree.

6.3

Accepted answers

(a) Osteomalacia (100%)
    Vitamin D deficiency (25%)

(b) Malabsorption (100%)
    Dietary deficiency (100%)
    Alcohol abuse (100%)
    Vitamin B_{12} and folate deficiency (100%)

(c) Vitamin D
    Calcium supplements

Osteomalacia is suggested by the low calcium and phosphate and the raised alkaline phosphatase.

Osteomalacia used to be common in Asian immigrants to Britain due to a combination of factors such as calcium binding by phytate in chapattis (leavened bread), decreased intake (many Asians are vegans), decreased synthesis of endogenous vitamin D and decreased sunlight exposure. Chapatti flour is now supplemented with calcium and vitamin D.

Causes of osteomalacia and rickets will be discussed further in a later question.

6.4

Accepted answers

(a) Congenital syphilis

(b) IgM fluorescent treponemal antibody test

Explanation

We included this question because it demonstrates that you may be able to work out more than you think you know.

This child is sick. The possibilities are that he has a treponemal infection (most likely congenital syphilis) or that this is a 'false positive VDRL' associated with another symptomatic condition that he has acquired. Considering the causes of a positive VDRL, none except syphilis is likely to be associated with this clinical syndrome. This means that he is most likely to have congenital syphilis.

On the basis of the fact that IgM does not cross the placental barrier, any IgM detectable in the baby must be in response to an active infection. IgM synthesis does not normally begin until 6 months of age but in neonatal infections synthesis begins earlier. Hence the diagnosis is confirmed by requesting IgM fluorescent treponemal antibody (FTA) test.

Other neonatal infections to consider are toxoplasmosis, rubella, herpes simplex, CMV and HIV.

Causes of positive VDRL
● Infections
Syphilis
Yaws
Leptospirosis
Hepatitis A
EBV
Mycoplasma
Bacterial endocarditis
● Tropical disease
Leprosy
Malaria
Trypanosomiases
Filariasis
● Autoimmune diseases
SLE
Sjögren's disease
Hashimoto's thyroiditis
Haemolytic anaemia
● Old age

6.5

Accepted answers

(a) Multiple endocrine neoplasia, type 2 (MEN 2) (100%)
   Sipple's syndrome (100%)

   Syndrome of phaeochromocytoma, medullary carcinoma of thyroid and parathyroid
      hyperplasia (75%)

(b) Serum calcitonin assay (100%)
   Plasma catecholamines (100%)

(c) Medullary carcinoma of the thyroid (cause of diarrhoea unknown) (100%)
   Phaeochromocytoma (presumably due to catecholamine-induced sympathetic
      activity) (100%)
   Vasoactive intestinal peptide production (VIP) (may be a feature of MEN 2) (100%)

(d) Hyperparathyroidism
   Phaeochromocytoma may be associated with hypercalcaemia, even with normal parathyroid glands

Explanation

There are a number of multiple endocrine diseases, and MEN 1 and MEN 2 are particular favourites. MEN 1 consists of the three 'P' tumours: **p**ituitary adenomata, **p**arathyroid adenomata causing hypercalcaemia, and **p**ancreatic tumours of diverse types (most commonly insulinomas or gastrinomas). Any of these may dominate the clinical presentation. Other occasional features include thyroid disease, carcinoid tumours and multiple lipomata.

   MEN 2, often inherited, consists of medullary carcinoma of the thyroid, phaeochromocytoma and, frequently, parathyroid hyperplasia. Medullary carcinoma of the thyroid comprises only a small proportion of thyroid neoplasms, and usually presents either as a goitre or is found incidentally when screening patients suspected of having MEN 2. Even in the absence of other endocrine disease defining MEN 2, the tumour is often familial. The C-cells of the thyroid produce calcitonin, and serum levels can be used for screening family and to determine adequacy of surgical clearance, but the calcitonin appears to have no significant effect on calcium metabolism. Treatment is total thyroidectomy as the tumour is often multifocal.

Phaeochromocytoma

As in this patient, it may be part of MEN 2 (and patients should have calcitonin levels measured) but is also associated with neurofibromatosis. The clinical manifestations and stage at which the tumour presents depend in part on how far the catecholamines are metabolized prior to their release into the circulation. Thus, if adrenaline, with predominant β-receptor affinity, is the major metabolite, the hypertension may be predominantly systolic. Clues which the examiners may leave to suggest the diagnosis of phaeochromocytoma in the appropriate context include:

- Sustained rather than paroxysmal hypertension in 50%.
- Postural hypotension due to reduction in intravascular volume.
- Anxiety, fear and sweating with or after paroxysms.
- Palpitations.
- Paroxysms after particular movements, or after micturition in patients with bladder wall tumours.
- Impaired glucose tolerance – adrenaline inhibits the hepatic uptake of glucose.

Diagnostic tests are confounded by the large number of drugs and foods which interfere with catecholamine metabolism (methyldopa, tetracyclines, phenothiazines, banana, tea, coffee, vanilla, etc) and by their variable metabolism within the tumours themselves. The initial test is for urinary catecholamine metabolites (vanillylmandelic acid, metanephrines) with careful attention to diet and drugs. Plasma catecholamines can be measured by high pressure liquid chromatography but will be elevated by stress and exercise.

   Most tumours occur in the adrenal glands and most will be visualized by CT scanning. $[^{131}I]$-metaiodobenzylguanadine (MIBG) binds to the tumour and is being increasingly used to visualize it. If selective venous sampling is performed, α-blockade and then β-blockade is essential prior to the procedure which may provoke paroxysms. β-blockade protects against arrhythmias. Similar precautions are necessary before surgery. A popular question concerns those drugs which you would want on the anaesthetic trolley at surgery for a phaeochromocytoma. They are:

- Phentolamine and nitroprusside for control of blood pressure.
- Propanolol to protect the heart from the arrhythmogenic catecholamines.

- Isoprenaline and noradrenaline in case of excessive α-blockade.

It is clearly a better answer to recognize that these two tumours comprise a syndrome rather than naming them individually. Having made the diagnosis, serum calcitonin is the definitive investigation.

6.6

Accepted answers

(a) Patient 2

(b) He has previously been the recipient of a kidney sharing HLA antigens with the current donor

(c) Patient 1: Positive crossmatch
Patient 3: Mismatched blood group

(d) Pregnancy
Blood transfusion

Explanation

The contraindications for transplantation are always changing. Time was when late middle age was a contraindication, or diabetics were discriminated against. Now most units in the UK will exclude *a priori* only those patients who are likely to reject the kidney for immunological reasons.

Several steps are involved in choosing the most appropriate recipient for a renal transplant. Potential recipients are usually tested regularly for their antibody reactivity to a panel of different HLA antigens. High reactivity against this panel make it unlikely that a donor kidney will become available which will give a negative cross-match, and this is often considered a contraindication to transplantation in itself. Unfortunately some patients have persistent high reactivity, usually due to previous multiple blood transfusions, previous pregnancies or previous transplantation. Some units are attempting to deal with these patients by adsorbing out their antibodies in

advance of transplantation. Fortunately, recombinant erythropoeitin is reducing the need for blood transfusion in end-stage renal failure.

Once a donor kidney becomes available, it is usually matched to the most appropriate recipient. First, the blood group of the donor is compared with those of the potential recipients; ABO incompatibility between donor and recipient is an absolute contraindication. Once a suitable recipient is chosen, a crossmatch is performed to detect whether the recipient has antibodies (predominantly anti-HLA antibodies) to donor cells. A positive crossmatch is correlated with the antibody-mediated hyperacute rejection and is a contraindication to transplantation.

The issue of HLA matching is controversial. Some units argue that in the age of cyclosporin, there is insufficient additional advantage to justify the constraints of HLA matching. Those who do favour matching try to match at three loci if possible (HLA-A, HLA-B and HLA-DR). This approach gives a maximum of six out of six exact HLA antigen matches, as most individuals have two alleles at each loci. An additional problem is whether to transplant a kidney into a recipient who has had a previous transplant which shared HLA antigens with the new donor graft. One might expect the patient to have been sensitized to these antigens and therefore have a positive crossmatch with the new donor cells. In fact, the crossmatch can be negative, but the patient may still develop an antibody response once the second kidney is transplanted. Although this is a potential problem, it may be reasonable

to proceed. In fact, this patient lost his first kidney within the first 24 h (for mechanical reasons).

The final issue is of recurrence in the transplant of the disease that destroyed the native kidneys. This occurs in several conditions, but is not usually considered as a contraindication to transplantation. Anti-GBM disease is a special consideration, since, unlike the others, it is self-limiting. Typically, once the acute illness has subsided and the anti-GBM antibody titre has remained low or absent for a suitable period (perhaps 6 months to 1 year), the patient can be considered for transplantation.

6.7

Accepted answers

(a) Hyper-osmolar non-ketotic diabetic coma

(b) Intravenous fluid replacement with hypotonic saline
Restoration of normoglycaemia with intravenous insulin
Anticoagulation with heparin

Explanation

Hyper-osmolar non-ketotic diabetic coma presents most frequently in the elderly. These patients have no ketones in the urine or blood, are not acidotic and thus do not hyperventilate. Often there is an insidious onset over weeks. The majority of patients are not comatose, but confused or stuporose. They may present with focal neurological signs. The blood glucose is very high (around 60 mmol/l), resulting in an osmotic diuresis in which large amounts of water, potassium and sodium are lost. Water loss is greatest, so the serum sodium is usually raised. This combination of

raised sodium and glucose gives a high serum osmolality. Pre-renal ureamia results from fluid depletion.

As fluid loss is severe, this must be replaced, usually with hypotonic saline if the sodium is very high (above 155 mmol/l). Potassium supplements should be given (10 mmol/h is usually adequate). Blood glucose should be normalized with insulin, as for the management of ketoacidosis. As the risk of thrombosis is significantly increased, anticoagulation should be considered. Finally, an underlying or precipitating cause, such as pancreatitis or infection, should be sought.

6.8

Accepted answers

(a) Small intestinal lymphangiectasia

(b) Small intestinal biopsy
     Barium studies of the small bowel
     Faecal excretion of intravenously
     administered $^{51}CrCl_3$

Rejected answer

Protein-losing enteropathy

Explanation

In this case, the differential diagnosis can be centred around causes of hypoalbuminaemia. These are malnutrition (and malignancy), liver failure, renal failure or protein-losing entero-pathy. Malnutrition is unlikely, the liver function tests are normal and there is no other evidence to suggest liver failure, and nephrotic syndrome is ruled out by the lack of protein-uria. This leaves a protein-losing enteropathy, causes of which are shown below.

In this case, the key to diagnosis is the lymphopenia and immunoglobulin deficiency, which is characteristic of small intestinal lymphangiectasia. This rare condition may present at any time, but is most common in the first few years of life. The pathological feature is dilatation of lymphatic channels, rupture of which is thought to cause hypo-proteinaemia and lymphocyte loss. The con-dition may be primary, but it has also been described as a secondary condition associated with other disorders such as constrictive pericarditis. The primary abnormality may be associated with lymphatic abnormalities out-side of the intestine, but may also be confined to the small bowel.

Clinical presentation may be with diarrhoea or steatorrhoea, hypoproteinaemia and oedema, recurrent infection, or, in childhood, failure to thrive. A firm diagnosis is made by establishing lymphatic abnormalities on small intestinal biopsy; however, lesions may be intermittent along the course of the bowel and thus a negative biopsy may not necessarily exclude the diagnosis. Barium studies typically show coarse mucosal folds. Radioisotopic techniques may demonstrate abnormal enteric loss of protein; intravenous $^{51}CrCl_3$ is most commonly used. Management consists of dietary manipulation to reduce the amount of long-chain fat which is usually absorbed via the small intestinal lymphatics. This in turn reduces pressure in the dilated lymphatics. Surgical resection may be possible if the lesions are localized.

Causes of enteric protein loss
Neoplastic disorders
    Gastric or colonic tumours
    Lymphoma
Inflammatory and infectious disorders
    Ulcerative colitis
    Crohn's disease
    Coeliac disease
    Tropical sprue
    Intestinal infections or infestations
    Postinfective ·
Lymphatic disorders
    Idiopathic small intestinal lymphangiect-
       asia
    Secondary lymphangiectasia
       Cardiac or pericardial disease
       Abdominal malignancy
       Tuberculous lymphadenitis
Whipple's disease
Giant rugae of stomach (Menetrier's disease)
Villous adenoma of colon
Fistulae and diverticulae

6.9

Accepted answer

Carbon tetrachloride poisoning

Explanation

A massively raised AST in excess of 25,000 IU/l is characteristic of liver necrosis secondary to **carbon tetrachloride toxicity**. Although carbon tetrachloride was once used as a dry cleaning agent, it is now limited to industrial use. Exposure to low concentrations may cause fatty degeneration of the liver; higher concentrations will cause centrilobular necrosis and necrosis of renal tubules.

Acute exposure is followed by nausea, vomiting, diarrhoea and abdominal pain. High concentrations can lead to confusion and coma; death may result if exposure is not terminated. Typically, liver damage is maximal 2 days after exposure and may progress to fulminant hepatic failure and encephalopathy. Acute tubular necrosis is the result of direct toxicity and may occur in the absence of hepatic dysfunction. Hepatic enzyme levels rise in advance of jaundice.

Individuals appear to differ in their sensitivity to carbon tetrachloride. Previous hepatic or renal disease or high alcohol consumption, as in this case, may increase susceptibility.

Early administration of *N*-acetylcysteine may be of benefit, but otherwise management is that of liver and renal failure, including dialysis when appropriate.

6.10

Accepted answers

(a) Stress polycythaemia (100%)
     Pseudopolycythaemia (100%)
     Relative polycythaemia (100%)
     Gaisböck's syndrome (100%)

(b) None

Rejected answers

Polycythaemia rubra vera
Any cause of secondary polycythaemia

The patient has a raised haemoglobin and red cell count. These are both expressed as a concentration. The red cell mass is normal; therefore the plasma volume must be decreased. This means the diagnosis must be pseudopolycythaemia.

There are other clues that exclude other diagnoses. Given the clinical setting and normal blood gases, it is reasonable (in the examination) to exclude all the secondary causes of polycythaemia. Similarly, with normal white cell and platelet counts and no features of myeloproliferative disease, there is no suggestion of polycythaemia rubra vera. (A lone raised RBC may be an early preneoplastic condition, in which case it is called benign (or idiopathic) erythrocytosis.)

Pseudopolycythaemia is a poorly defined condition in which the red cell mass tends to the upper limit of normal, the plasma volume tends to the lower limit of normal and hence haemoglobin and red cell counts are elevated. Individuals with this condition tend to be middle-aged obese men with mild hypertension. There is a debate about whether or not this condition is associated with an increased risk of cerebrovascular and coronary artery disease. For the time being there is no indication for treatment of an otherwise asymptomatic individual.

Causes of polycythaemia

True polycythaemia
- Primary
    Polycythaemia rubra vera
    Benign (idiopathic) erythrocytosis
- Secondary
    Chronic hypoxia
        Altitude
        Lung disease
        Cyanotic congenital heart disease
        Haemoglobinopathies
        Decreased production of 2,3-DPG
    Inappropriately high erythropoietin secretion
        Renal pathology
            Tumour
            Cyst
            Hydronephrosis
            Post-renal transplant
        Other tumours
            Hepatoma
            Cerebellar haemangioblastoma
            Uterine fibroma
        Genetic abnormality of erythropoietin control
    Endocrine (mechanism unknown)
        Cushing's disease
        Phaeochromocytoma

Pseudopolycythaemia
(Synonyms: stress polycythaemia, relative polycythaemia, Gaisböck's syndrome)

Answers to Data Interpretation Paper 7

7.1

Accepted answers

(a) Inferior myocardial infarction and complete heart block

(b) Occlusion of the right coronary artery resulting in ischaemia of the atrioventricular node (100%)

Occlusion of the dominant circumflex artery resulting in ischaemia of the atrioventricular node (100%)

(c) Observation

(d) The patient is asymptomatic (has a normal blood pressure)

Rejected answers

Cardiac pacing

Medical therapy (atropine, adrenaline)

The patient is in complete heart block

Explanation

The examiners expect comprehensive knowledge of common medical emergencies. It is important to be aware of basic coronary artery anatomy as this explains both the site of infarction and some of the complications. Both the inferior myocardium and the artery to the AV node are supplied by the right coronary artery or by a dominant circumflex artery. The correct answer to (c) and (d) is observation as the patient is asymptomatic. The block is often temporary but normal conduction may not be restored for 2 weeks.

The question also re-emphasizes the need for complete answers. Incomplete answers attract lower marks or are rejected.

Other important complications of myocardial infarction recognizable on the ECG include:

- AV block in anterior infarction suggests very extensive infarction.
- Atrial fibrillation.
- Ventricular tachyarrhythmias.
- Ventricular aneurysm, more common after anterior than inferior infarction.

Indications for temporary pacing

Following acute myocardial infarction (MI)
   Only if cardiac output impaired (i.e. low blood pressure, confused)
   Anterior MI
      Complete heart block
      Second-degree heart block
      Alternating left and right bundle branch block
      Right bundle branch block and left axis deviation
   Post asystolic cardiac arrest
Other indications
   Symptomatic bradycardia or sinus arrest not reversed by atropine
   Complete heart block
   Second degree heart block ⎫ if symptomatic
   Pauses   ⎬ with dizziness
   Bradycardia   ⎭ or syncope
   Prior to cardiac surgery
   Prior to general anaesthesia if complete heart block or second-degree heart block
   In selected situations when using anti-arrhythmic drugs

7.2

Accepted answers

(a) Acquired sideroblastic anaemia

(b) Bone marrow examination for ring sideroblasts

Explanation

The key points in this case are: a raised MCV, which is often seen in acquired (but not hereditary) sideroblastic anaemia; a raised serum iron and ferritin; and a mixed normo-chromic/hypochromic blood film, characteristic of sideroblastic anaemia.

The hereditary form usually occurs in males. Splenomegaly is unusual in the acquired form, but can occur. Platelet levels are reduced in 30% of patients with acquired disease, but may occasionally be raised.

> **Causes of acquired sideroblastic anaemia**
> Primary
> Myeloproliferative disease
> Drugs (e.g. antituberculous drugs)
> Lead
> Alcohol

7.3

Accepted answers

(a) Intestinal lymphoma

(b) Alpha-chain disease (100%)
Whipple's disease (100%)
Intestinal tuberculosis (100%)
Crohn's disease (100%)

(c) Jejunal biopsy (100%)
Gastric washings for mycobacteria (100%)
Lymph node excision/biopsy (100%)

Rejected answers

Fulminant liver failure

Fulminant liver failure

Barium studies
Hydrogen breath test
Abdominal ultrasound

Explanation

The data strongly suggest biliary obstruction, but the marked hypoalbuminaemia suggests disease of the intestinal mucosa in addition. Because of the lymphadenopathy, lympho-cytosis and hint of intermittent fever, the likely diagnosis is a lymphoma of the intestine with obstructive jaundice due to nodes at the porta hepatis. The only diagnostic test is tissue biopsy, although ultrasound will confirm biliary obstruction and the appearances of a barium meal and follow-through may be characteristic.

Alpha-chain disease is an immunoproliferative disorder of plasmacytoid cells of the small intestine, producing incomplete heavy chains of IgA. They may undergo malignant transformation to a lymphoma. A lymphoma would also be suggested by a history of dermatitis herpetiformis.

Whipple's disease is a rare infectious disease

tending to occur in middle-aged Europeans with polyarthritis, malabsorption, lymphadenopathy, fever, skin pigmentation and neurological disease both peripheral and central. It is characterized by macrophages containing a bacillus in the lamina propria of the intestinal mucosa. These have still not been definitively identified, but disappear slowly, along with resolution of the disease, on treatment with antibiotics. It is a rare Membership-type disease, but there is insufficient clinical evidence to support the diagnosis here.

It is important to consider the acquired immunodeficiency syndrome, where numerous pathogens may cause malabsorption although an aetiological agent in the gut may not be identified. The multisystem manifestations of the disease make it a consideration here, but some risk factor is likely to be specified.

A guide to malabsorption is given in the answer to Data Interpretation question 2.4.

7.4

Accepted answers	*Rejected answers*
(a) Blood glucose (100%) Urinalysis to detect glycosuria (100%)	
(b) Cranial diabetes insipidus	Diabetes insipidus Nephrogenic diabetes insipidus
(c) The plasma osmolality rose to 299 mOsm/kg	

Explanation

The water deprivation test is straightforward in principle. It is essentially a hormone stimulation test performed when there is a suspicion of a functional deficit of antidiuretic hormone (vasopressin; ADH), just as the Synacthen test is used in Addison's disease. The test is performed in two parts. In the first part, water deprivation is used as the stimulus to assess the patient's ability to produce ADH; in the second part, ADH is given (in the form of DDAVP) to assess the patient's ability to respond appropriately. In both parts the presence of effective ADH is determined by an ability to concentrate urine and thus increase urinary osmolality.

In theory, the interpretation of the test is also straightforward:

Urinary concentration in response to water deprivation	Urinary concentration in response to exogenous ADH	Diagnosis
+	+	Psychogenic polydipsia
−	+	Cranial diabetes insipidus
−	−	Nephrogenic diabetes insipidus

If there is normal urine concentration in both parts of the test, the diagnosis is primary polydipsia. The absence of a concentrating response to water deprivation (the first part) is diagnostic of diabetes insipidus (DI). If the second part is normal, you can conclude that the patient will respond to ADH, but is just not producing it himself: this is cranial diabetes insipidus. If the second part is also abnormal (i.e. he still fails to concentrate urine), you can conclude that his kidneys are unable to respond to ADH: this is nephrogenic diabetes insipidus.

In practice, however, there are complicating factors:

- There may be inadequate stimulus to ADH release; therefore, the test includes measurement of plasma osmolality. This must rise to at least 290 mOsm/kg for the stimulus to ADH to be adequate. For this reason it is important to continue with the first part of the test, i.e. the water deprivation for as long as possible. Since this can be dangerous, it is essential to weigh the patient hourly and discontinue the test if the weight falls by more than 3%.
- There may not be an adequate concentration gradient in the renal parenchyma because of prolonged polyuria. This would make urinary osmolality a poor index of ADH function. If adequate urinary concentration does occur at any stage in the test, then this cannot be a problem. If the urine does not concentrate at any point, then one cannot exclude an inadequate concentration gradient and the test may be difficult to interpret. In other words, the diagnosis of nephrogenic diabetes insipidus is difficult to make with certainty.
- In cranial diabetes insipidus there may only be a partial deficit of ADH release. In this case there may be some concentration in the

first part of the test. There is usually an obvious step-up in concentrating ability with the administration of DDAVP, which does not occur in patients without diabetes insipidus. However, in mild cranial diabetes insipidus, this may be difficult to interpret with confidence in a specific case.

In these situations one may be left with equivocal results. Clearly any test must be interpreted in its clinical context, but if doubt remains, a hypertonic saline challenge test may be used to increase the serum osmolality and correlate it with measured ADH levels. In the Examination, unless you are specifically asked a question about the reliability of your conclusions, assume that a failure to concentrate urine in response to water deprivation and DDAVP is diagnostic of nephrogenic DI.

In this particular question the patient could be polyuric because of steroid-induced diabetes mellitus. Hence the initial investigation should be a blood glucose. Alternatively, he could have cranial diabetes insipidus or hypothalamic polydipsia due to cerebral lymphoma; or he could have nephrogenic diabetes insipidus because his manic-depressive illness is being treated with lithium. Everything depends upon the water deprivation test which offers the correct diagnosis of cranial diabetes insipidus, caused in this case by a retro-orbital mass of lymphomatous tissue which had spread posteriorly.

7.5

Accepted answers

(a) Addison's disease (100%)

ACTH deficiency (75%)

(b) Tuberculosis

Explanation

Sodium depletion is the major biochemical abnormality resulting from adrenocorticoid hypofunction. When hyponatraemia occurs in

the presence of haemoconcentration (raised urea and creatinine) and hypoglycaemia, candidates must think of this diagnosis. Acute adrenal insufficiency is marked by hypotension and shock. Chronic insufficiency often results in postural hypotension. Other symptoms of chronic insufficiency include weight loss, malaise, vomiting, diarrhoea and non-specific abdominal pain.

It is difficult to distinguish primary adrenal insufficiency (Addison's disease) from ACTH deficiency. Pigmentation, which suggests Addison's disease, may be absent in those with autoimmune disease. ACTH deficiency is most commonly the result of exogenous steroid therapy. Otherwise, it occurs as part of generalized pituitary and hypothalamic disease. Spontaneous isolated ACTH deficiency is very rare, as is Sheehan's syndrome (pituitary infarction during pregnancy).

Hypoglycaemia (especially fasting) is caused by the absence of glucocorticoids. Other abnormalities include a raised plasma potassium and a metabolic acidosis.

In the West, the commonest form of Addison's is autoimmune. Rarer causes include amyloidosis and disseminated malignancy. However, tuberculosis used to be the most common cause and this must be seriously considered in high-risk individuals, such as the patient in this case. Because of the increased probability of tuberculosis, you would be awarded more marks for a diagnosis of Addison's than ACTH deficiency.

7.6

Accepted answers

(a) Pyloric stenosis

(b) Gastroscopy
   Barium meal

Explanation

The patient has a high plasma bicarbonate, low plasma potassium and low plasma chloride. The raised bicarbonate means the acid–base disturbance is either a metabolic alkalosis or a compensated respiratory acidosis. The low potassium favours metabolic alkalosis, which is caused by a primary rise in plasma bicarbonate.

In this case the likely diagnosis is pyloric stenosis. The hypochloraemia reflects gastric loss of chloride, which may result in a plasma chloride up to 80 mmol/l lower than plasma sodium (compared to the usual 40 mmol/l). Hypokalaemia results from the absence of hydrogen ions to compete for potassium secretion in the distal tubules of the kidney. Severe hypochloraemic alkalosis is now rare because pyloric stenosis is usually detected earlier.

> **Causes of a metabolic alkalosis**
> Ingestion or infusion of alkali
>   Sodium bicarbonate ingestion
>   Forced alkaline diuresis (e.g. for salicylate overdose)
>   Excess ingestion of alkali during therapy for acidosis
>   Milk–alkali syndrome
> Pyloric stenosis
> Persistent self-induced vomiting
> Potassium depletion (except tubular acidosis)
> Chloride depletion
> Hyperaldosteronism
> Fulminant liver failure

7.7

Accepted answers	*Rejected answer*
(a) Alcohol-induced hypertriglyceridaemia	
(b) Serum γGT (100%)	MCV
Blood alcohol level (50%)	

Explanation

The examiners are tempting you to think of primary hyperlipidaemias, but the isolated hypertriglyceridaemia with a normal cholesterol level forces you to consider secondary hyperlipidaemia (see table below). The most common cause of secondary hypertriglycerolaemla is alcohol abuse. In most hypertriglyceridaemic states, HDL cholesterol levels are low. The existence of a high triglyceride and raised HDL cholesterol, as in this case, strongly suggests alcohol lipaemia, although it may also be due to oestrogens. Note that HDL cholesterol is not always raised in alcohol induced lipaemia.

There is no conclusive laboratory test which will definitively demonstrate alcohol abuse. However, γ-glutamyl transferase is often elevated. A spot blood alcohol level may be of use, but will not indicate chronicity. As you are asked for a biochemical test, a raised MCV, which is a haematological parameter, would attract no marks.

Causes of hyperlipidaemia

Disorder	Hypercholesterolaemia	Hypertriglyceridaemia
Primary hyperlipidaemias		
Familial hypercholesterolaemia	+ + +	
Familial combined hyperlipidaemia	+	+
Familial hypertriglyceridaemia	+	+ + +
Lipoprotein lipase/apoC-II deficiency	+	+ + +
Remnant hyperlipoproteinaemia	+ +	+ +
Polygenic hypercholesterolaemia	+	
Secondary hyperlipidaemias		
Hypothyroidism	+	
Biliary obstruction	+	
Corticosteroids	+	
Diabetes mellitus		+
Alcohol excess		+
Chronic renal failure		+
Oral contraceptives		+
Thiazide diuretics		+
Nephrotic syndrome	+	+
Myeloma	+	+

7.8

Accepted answer

$$L^M L^M = 0.49$$
$$L^M L^N = 0.42$$
$$L^N L^N = 0.09$$

Explanation

Candidates often complain that Membership examinations (particularly Part 1) have little to do with the kind of medicine they deal with on a day to day basis. Questions can crop up which are completely outside the experience of most candidates. We would be surprised if you were asked a question on population genetics. Nevertheless we have included this question to illustrate that sometimes it is possible to answer questions from first principles, provided you have a clear mind. Unfortunately, clear minds are at a premium during the examination, so it pays to have a plan of action designed for this type of question. Remember, if the question is difficult, leave it until you have answered the other questions. You are then under less pressure and can think straighter.

To answer this question, first work out the frequencies of the two alleles L^M and L^N.

Blood group	Genotype	No. of individuals	No. of L^M alleles	No. of L^N alleles
M	$L^M L^M$	450	900	0
N	$L^M L^N$	500	500	500
N	$L^N L^N$	50	0	100
Total		1000	1400	600

The frequency of L^M, which we can call p, is $1400/2000 = 0.7$.
The frequency of L^N, which we can call q is $600/2000 = 0.3$.
Note that $p + q$ must equal 1.

During random mating, it can be assumed that the contribution of each allele to the next generation will reflect their frequency in the initial population, i.e. the ratio of LM gametes to LN gametes will be $0.7:0.3$. This ratio will be the same irrespective of whether the gamete is an egg or sperm. The next generation will thus be produced by the following mating combinations:

	L^M-bearing sperm (p = 0.7)	L^N-bearing sperm (q = 0.3)
L^M bearing eggs (p = 0.7)	$L^M L^M$ zygotes $p^2 = 0.49$	$L^M L^N$ zygotes $pq = 0.21$
L^N bearing eggs (p = 0.3)	$L^M L^N$ zygotes $pq = 0.21$	$L^N L^N$ zygotes $q^2 = 0.09$

The frequency of $L^M L^M$ genotypes will thus be $p^2 = 0.49$.
The frequency of $L^M L^N$ genotypes will thus be $2pq = 0.42$.
The frequency of $L^N L^N$ genotypes will thus be $q^2 = 0.09$.

Note that the allele frequencies in the new population are once again $p = 0.7$ and $q = 0.3$. Thus if this second generation population was to undergo random mating to produce a third generation, the genotype frequencies would be identical to the second generation! This is called Hardy–Weinberg equilibrium (HWE).

HWE is defined by a set of genotype frequencies p^2 of AA to $2pq$ of Aa to q^2 of aa, where A and a represent two alleles of a locus and p and q are the frequencies of A and a. If the ratio of AA:Aa:aa is p2:2pq:q2 then the population is in HWE. When this is the case, genotype and allele frequencies do not change from one generation to the next. In this question the genotype ratios of the initial population were $450:500:5$ ($L^M L^M : L^M L^N : L^N L^N$) whereas the ratio $p^2 : 2pq : q^2$ was $0.49:0.42:0.9$, so the population **was not** in HWE. But after one generation of random mating the genotype frequencies ($L^M L^M : L^M L^N : L^N L^N$) did equal $0.49 : 0.42 : 0.9$, so the next generation **was** in HWE.

This illustrates a principle of population genetics. If a population is not in Hardy–Weinberg equilibrium, then it takes only one generation of random mating to establish Hardy–Weinberg equilibrium.

Thus candidates who manage to remember this principle could quickly answer the question by working out the allele frequencies in the initial population (p and q) and realising that the genotype frequencies in the next population would be p^2, $2pq$ and q^2 – a process which should take under a minute. However, less fortunate candidates could still derive the answer by working it out in the manner shown above!

7.9

Accepted answer

Adverse interaction between allopurinol and azathioprine

Explanation

Allopurinol inhibits the enzyme xanthine oxidase which is involved in the production of uric acid from purines.

$$\text{Hypoxanthine} \xrightarrow[\text{oxidase}]{\text{Xanthine}} \text{Xanthine} \xrightarrow[\text{oxidase}]{\text{Xanthine}} \text{Uric acid}$$

Azathioprine has some therapeutic value itself, but is almost completely converted to 6-mercaptopurine. 6-Mercaptopurine is in turn metabolized to 6-thiouric acid by xanthine oxidase. For this reason, azathioprine require-ments are drastically reduced in the presence of allopurinol.

In this case, it is probable that the general practitioner unwittingly introduced allopurinol as a treatment for gout without altering the dose of azathioprine. The bone marrow depression caused by azathioprine increased and white blood cell count dropped.

Drug interactions provide a vast array of material on which questions can be based. The appendices in the British National Formulary provide a wealth of information on drug interactions, adverse reactions, etc. As many candidates carry the BNF around with them (or at least refer to it) every day, it pays to get into the habit of spending any spare time in the months prior to the Examination browsing through its appen-dices.

7.10

Accepted answers

  (a) Hookworm infestation
     Thalassaemia trait

  (b) Examination of blood film
     Iron studies (serum iron and iron binding capacity)
     Haemoglobin electrophoresis
     Microscopic examination of faecal smear

Rejected answers

Occult blood loss
Thalassaemia alpha or beta

Explanation

There is no excuse for getting this question wrong as a similar case was presented in Data Interpretation question 4.3! By now you should recognize that this question should be approached via the differential diagnosis of a microcytic anaemia. Abdominal pain in a child from the Mediterranean with microcytic anaemia is sufficient evidence to suggest chronic blood loss from hookworm infestation and thus iron deficient anaemia; it is estimated that hookworm is responsible for the loss of 700 l of blood per day around the world. The second likely cause in this patient is thalassaemia trait. Note there is insufficient data here to distinguish between α- and β-thalassaemia.

As previously discussed, plasma ferritin, total iron-binding capacity (TIBC), and marrow iron are measures of iron stores; in iron deficiency ferritin and marrow iron fall while TIBC rises. In thalassaemia they are normal or may indicate increased iron stores. The blood film is the most basic and simplest of investigations; although it may not be possible to distinguish iron deficiency and thalassaemia trait, pencil cells and anisocytosis are more pronounced in the former and target cells in the latter.

The thalassaemias are a popular subject because the data tests your understanding of basic pathophysiology. What follows is a greatly simplified summary of the essential information. Most adult haemoglobin is HbA, consisting of two β chains and two α chains. Fetal haemoglobin, HbF, has two α and two γ chains. A small proportion of adult haemoglobin is HbA2, with α and δ chains. β-Thalassaemia major is where there is deletion or mutation of both β genes; the proportion of HbF rises to compensate and there is transfusion-dependent anaemia with haemolysis. These patients often develop transfusion-induced haemochromatosis. In β-thalassaemia trait, only one β gene is absent (i.e. the patient is heterozygous) and there is mild hypochromic anaemia, as here, with slight elevations of HbA2 and HbF.

Two α chain genes exist, α1 and α2, giving a total of four per individual, any number of which may be absent. Single gene deletions are usually clinically silent. Two gene deletions results in α-thalassaemia trait, with the same haematological picture as its β counterpart. Haemoglobin H disease results from triple gene deletion; there is variable anaemia with splenomegaly and a typical thalassaemia blood picture. Deletion of all four genes is incompatible with life as α chains are a component of all three major haemoglobin types.

Haemoglobin electrophoresis at an alkaline pH allows the proportions of HbA, HbA2 and HbF to be determined and hence the likely diagnosis, e.g. HbA2 is typically elevated in beta thalassaemia trait but not alpha trait. However, a definitive diagnosis requires a globin chain synthesis study.

Answers to Data Interpretation Paper 8

8.1

Accepted answer

Hypertrophic cardiomyopathy

Explanation

The M-mode echocardiographic features of hypertrophic cardiomyopathy are:

- Asymmetrical hypertrophy of the septum compared to the posterior free wall of the left ventricle (seen in this case).
- The mitral valve appears to fill the left ventricle (seen in this case).

- Systolic anterior movement ('SAM') of the mitral anterior valve leaflet on to the septum (not seen so well in this case).

A guide to M-mode echocardiography is given in the answer to Data Interpretation question 2.2.

8.2

Accepted answers

(a) Systemic lupus erythematosus
Pre-eclampsia

(b) Anti-double stranded DNA antibody titre
Anti-nuclear factor antibody titre
Serum complement levels

Rejected answers

Glomerulonephritis

Renal biopsy
Plasma urate

Explanation

The diagnosis of pre-eclampsia can be difficult, as other disorders, including malignant hypertension, produce similar clinical pictures. The final proof that the diagnosis of pre-eclampsia is correct comes following delivery, at which point it disappears, while other conditions persist. This alone is evidence that pre-eclampsia is a distinct condition associated with the gravid uterus, different from other causes of hypertension in pregnancy.

Pre-eclampsia is the most common cause of nephrotic syndrome during pregnancy. One of its earliest signs is an increase in plasma urate. Proteinurea is a relatively late sign, as is an increase in plasma urea and creatinine. Hypertension is also an early feature and, of course,

must be present for the diagnosis to be made. Although 85% of pre-eclamptics have oedema, this is not necessary for a positive diagnosis. Headaches, abdominal pain and vomiting suggest that progression to eclampsia is imminent.

The major differential in this case is SLE, which can be difficult to distinguish from pre-eclampsia. A positive VDRL would favour the diagnosis of SLE, as antiphospholipid antibodies (lupus anticoagulant), which give a false-positive VDRL, are commonly found in SLE. Afro-Caribbeans also have a higher risk of developing SLE. However, yaws may be an alternative cause of the positive VDRL. Pre-eclampsia is not associated with the skin, joint and pleuritic symptoms of SLE. High titres of anti-nuclear factor and anti-double stranded DNA antibody, and low serum complement levels further support the diagnosis of SLE. Although renal biopsy would distinguish between the two conditions, it is not indicated as delivery of the child will treat the putative pre-eclampsia.

Other forms of glomerulonephritis occasionally present for the first time during pregnancy and can be difficult to distinguish from pre-eclampsia. Once again, delivery of the child will aid diagnosis and, of course, treatment.

Causes of a positive VDRL are discussed in the answer to Data Interpretation question 6.4.

8.3

Accepted answers

(a) Right sided low-tone deafness

(b) Ménière's disease

Explanation

The diagnosis of Ménière's disease is based on a classical history of fluctuation of the characteristic features: sensorineural deafness, tinnitus, vertigo (typically lasting hours) and a feeling of fullness in the affected ear. The approach to audiograms is discussed in the answer to Data Interpretation question 4.9.

8.4

Accepted answer

Hyperkalaemia

Rejected answers

Metabolic acidosis
Renal failure
Ketoacidosis

Explanation

The ECG shows the typical abnormalities associated with hyperkalaemia: peaked, tall T waves, widened QRS complexes and diminution of P wave amplitude.

As you are asked for the cause of the ECG abnormalities, the correct answer is **hyperkalaemia**. An answer which gives one of the **causes of hyperkalaemia** would be incorrect.

A discussion on non-cardiac ECG abnormalities can be found in the answer to Data Interpretation question 3.2.

8.5

Accepted answers	*Rejected answer*
(a) Obstructive defect: low FEV_1/FVC Destruction of alveolar walls: low TL_{CO} and K_{CO} and increased TLC	
(b) Histiocytosis X (100%)	Letterer–Siwe disease
Hand–Schuller–Christian disease (90%) Eosinophilic granuloma (90%)	
Neurofibromatosis (75%) Tuberous sclerosis (75%)	
Lymphangio(leio)myomatosis (25%)	

Explanation

These diseases share a potential to cause widespread cystic change in the lung, with a predisposition to pneumothoraces. In histiocytosis X, infiltration by histiocytes and other cells produces a pattern of pulmonary function mimicking pulmonary fibrosis, but as cystic changes develop the pattern described above develops. Apart from the rarity of the other pulmonary diseases named, the polyuria suggests possible diabetes insipidus due to posterior pituitary histiocytic granulomata, which is why histiocytosis X is the best answer. Histiocytosis X occurs in three forms: eosinophilic granuloma, Hand–Schuller–Christian disease and Letterer–Siwe disease. The last presents in childhood. Lymphangio(leio)myomatosis is extremely uncommon in males. Causes of emphysema in a young patient (i.e. α_1-antitrypsin deficiency) are effectively ruled out by the appearance of the chest X-ray.

8.6

Accepted answers	*Rejected answers*
(a) Vitamin D-resistant rickets (100%) X-linked hypophosphataemic rickets (synonym) (100%)	Vitamin D-dependent rickets Osteomalacia
(b) Widened epiphyseal growth plate (100%) Fraying, splaying and cupping of metaphysis (100%) Indistinct cortex due to poorly calcified underlying osteoid (100%) Cupping of anterior ends of ribs giving rachitic rosary (100%) Tendon calcification (100%)	
(c) 24-hour urinary phosphate estimation	Serum vitamin D levels
(d) The daughters will	Yes No

Explanation

Rickets (osteomalacia in adults) is a disease of inadequate bone mineralization. This is usually due to vitamin D deficiency or abnormalities of its metabolism, but it also occurs as a result of increased renal clearance of phosphate and hence hypophosphataemia.

Causes of rickets and osteomalacia
- Vitamin D disorders
  - Dietary deficiency
  - Inadequate absorption
  - Disorders of metabolism
    - Hereditary (vitamin D-dependent rickets)
    - Anticonvulsants
    - Renal failure
- Renal loss of phosphate
  - Chronic acidosis (e.g. renal tubular acidosis, acetazolamide)
  - Hereditary renal phosphate leak
    - Vitamin D-resistant rickets
    - Neurofibromatosis
  - Generalized tubular disorders (Fanconi's syndrome, e.g. Wilson's disease, myeloma)
- Primary mineralization defects (rare)
  - Hereditary hypophosphatasia
  - Etidronate treatment

If the patient has one of the vitamin D disorders you are likely to be given a clue to abnormal vitamin D metabolism, e.g. the patient is vegan or on anticonvulsants.

In addition it is often possible to distinguish vitamin D disorders from hypophosphataemic states biochemically: serum calcium is normally depressed in the vitamin D group, and normal in the phosphate-losing group. However, this is not invariably true. Hypophosphataemia occurs in both groups: in the vitamin D group, secondary hyperparathyroidism enhances renal phosphate loss.

Vitamin D-resistant rickets is an X-linked hereditary disorder of renal phosphate handling with no other renal abnormality except an increase in urinary glycine. There is an associated inappropriately low level of 1,25-dihydroxyvitamin D (1,25(OH)$_2$-vitamin D), and patients respond to combined phosphorus and vitamin D supplementation. Calcification or ossification of tendon insertions, ligaments and joint capsules is a unique feature of this disorder.

Vitamin D-dependent rickets is another rare form useful for the examination as it tests your understanding of vitamin D metabolism. In type 1, there is a low level of 1,25(OH)$_2$-vitamin D due to a defect in renal hydroxylation, so that the biochemistry is difficult to distinguish from dietary rickets unless the 25-hydroxyvitamin D level is known. This is the metabolite measured in most 'vitamin D' assays. The disease has an autosomal recessive inheritance.

In type 2 vitamin D-dependent rickets there is resistance to the effects of 1,25(OH)$_2$-vitamin D, the levels of which are therefore elevated. At a molecular level, this is a spectrum of disorders with several different mechanisms of resistance. Alopecia may be associated with the bony abnormalities. High doses of vitamin D are required for treatment.

8.7

Accepted answers

The patient has gone from lying to standing between the two tests (100%)
The first sample is taken uncuffed, the second sample cuffed (100%)

Venous stasis (50%)

Rejected answers

Laboratory error
Normal biological variation
Normal variability in test results
First specimen taken from same arm as IV drip

Explanation

With the exception of the sodium and potassium (which remain essentially unchanged), all the values have increased. It is unlikely that random biological or laboratory variation would push all results in the same direction. In fact there is mild haemoconcentration. This is the result of the increased venous pressure that occurs on standing up. Cells, proteins and protein-bound substances are retained while solutes leach out with the fluid.

An alternative cause of venous hypertension might be local venous stasis. However, if this occurs for any period of time hypoxia results in loss of potasisum from within the cells.

An alternative to haemoconcentration of the second sample might be haemodilution of the first. However, if there is a drip running into the arm, one can expect a rise in one or more of the glucose, sodium or albumin.

8.8

Accepted answers

(a) Paroxysmal nocturnal haemoglobinuria

(b) Ham test

Explanation

This patient has the characteristic laboratory findings of paroxysmal nocturnal haemoglobinuria (PNH); neutropenia, anaemia, thrombocytopenia and reticulocytosis. The diagnosis can be based upon the differential diagnosis of neutropenia, discussed in the answer to Data Interpretation question 5.5. PNH is an acquired clonal disease, thought to arise from a somatic mutation affecting the cell membrane. It affects leucocytes, platelets and red cells. The abnormality of the red cell membrane renders it sensitive to lysis by complement, resulting in a chronic intravascular haemolysis.

PNH typically presents between the ages of 20 and 40 in both males and females. Patients often present with gradual onset of exertional dyspnoea and malaise, and occasionally slight jaundice. Characteristically, this is accompanied by the intermittent passage of dark urine due to haemoglobinuria. This often occurs mostly at night resulting in discolouration of the urine passed first thing in the morning. It is possible, however, for the haemoglobinuria to go unnoticed during the course of the disease.

The degree of the haematological abnormalities may vary. Anaemia may be severe enough to warrant transfusion. Reticulocyte counts vary from less than 1% to 40%, and neutrophil and platelet counts can also vary widely. The blood film appearance may be unremarkable, and the MCV may be high, reflecting the reticulocytosis. The plasma contains free haemoglobin. Haptoglobins are typically absent and Hb electrophoresis normal.

The classic diagnostic laboratory test is the Ham test which involves suspending red cells in fresh normal ABO-compatible serum acidified to pH 6.5. The acidification activates the alternative complement pathway.

8.9

Accepted answers   *Rejected answers*

(a) Antiphospholipid syndrome (100%)
     Lupus anticoagulant (100%)
     Anticardiolipin antibodies (100%)

(b) Antiphospholipid antibody titre (100%)

     APTT assay using mixture of patients
       serum and normal plasma (75%)

     VDRL (10%)

(c) Aspirin therapy   Antiphospholipid syndrome
                                                  Lupus anticoagulant
                                                  Anticardiolipin antibodies

Explanation

The lupus anticoagulant (LA) is an *in vitro* inhibitor of phospholipid-dependent coagulation assays which was first described in patients with systemic lupus erythematosis. LA activity is believed to be due to an antibody against the phospholipid component of the prothrombinase complex, which cleaves prothrombin to form thrombin. It is associated with high titres of anticardiolipin antibodies and a false-positive test for syphilis.

Individuals with raised anticardiolipin (aCL) antibodies or LA have an increased risk of arterial and venous thrombosis, thrombocytopenia and recurrent abortion. The association of clinical manifestations with raised aCL antibodies or LA has been termed the antiphospholipid syndrome. Thirty to forty per cent of SLE patients have aCL antibodies, but they have also been detected in a number of other disorders, including migraine, malignancy, autoimmune thrombocytopenia, myasthaenia gravis, and multiple sclerosis. They are also found in patients with vascular disease, e.g. following myocardial infarction or stroke. Patients with cerebral ischaemia associated with aCL antibodies tend to be younger and have recurrent vascular events.

Diagnosis is made on the basis of abnormal coagulation tests and the detection of aCL antibodies. Typically the activated partial thromboplastin time is prolonged and cannot be corrected by mixing with plasma, indicating the presence of an inhibitor rather than the absence of clotting factors. The prothrombin time is usually normal or slightly prolonged. The bleeding time, a measure of platelet function, is normal – in this case it is abnormal because the patient has taken aspirin.

8.10

Accepted answer

Pregnancy

Explanation

We end the data interpretation section with an example of an old favourite which is neverthe-less worth repeating – seemingly abnormal values which are in fact due to the physiological changes of pregnancy. In a woman of child-bearing age, always keep pregnancy in mind if the diagnosis seems obscure.

Physiological changes in pregnancy

Cardiovascular
   Blood volume (plasma volume and red cell volume) increases
   Cardiac output increases
   Peripheral resistance falls
Endocrine
   Increased throxine-binding globulin
   Increased levels of T3 and T4 (but free T3 and T4 remain in the normal range)
   Increased peripheral resistance to insulin
   Increased tendency to glycosuria
Haematological
   Red cell mass increases
   Haemoglobin concentration, packed cell volume and red cell count fall (Hb may fall further
      if iron deficiency also occurs)
   MCV rises slightly
   Platelet count may increase, but may also fall due to haemodilution
   Serum ferritin falls
   Blood viscosity falls
   Concentrations of factors VII, VIII and X and fibrinogen increase
Renal
   Renal blood flow and glomerular filtration increase
   Clearance of urea, urate, creatinine increases (and plasma levels fall)
Respiratory
   Tidal volume increases
   $PaCO_2$ and plasma bicarbonate fall
Immunological
   Serum immunoglobulin concentrations fall

SECTION 3

SECTION 3 – PICTORIAL MATERIAL

In preparing for this section, try to see as many examples as possible prior to the examination. Even more than in the Case Histories section, in this part of the examination almost anything can be shown; so breadth of knowledge is important.

However, like the data interpretation, it is possible to predict some of what you will be shown. Common investigations such as chest X-rays and bone marrows are favourites. Prior to the examination you should prepare lists of the more common conditions likely to be presented to you. As we have said before, practise logical methods of looking at pictures (for example, of chest X-rays) for use when an abnormality is not immediately apparent. We will suggest these for certain classes of picture. In some examples, however, the answer is straightforward and simply depends upon pattern recognition.

In our examples, we have introduced a slight bias towards those areas candidates find particularly difficult, such as haematology, ophthalmology, and tropical medicine.

Pictorial Material Paper 1

1.1
a) Name three physical signs.
b) What is the likely diagnosis?

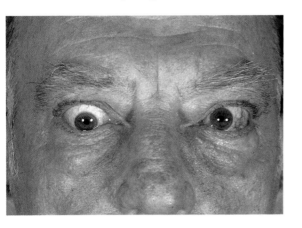

1.2
What is the diagnosis?

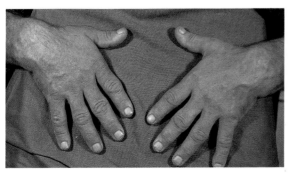

1.3
What is this papular eruption?

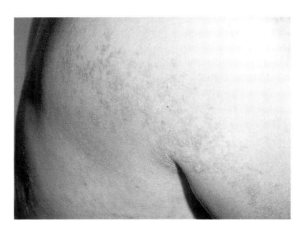

1.4
a) What are the abnormal cells?
b) What is the most likely diagnosis?

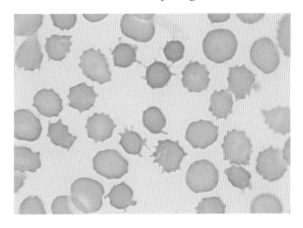

1.5
a) What is the complete diagnosis?
b) What are the two clinical features of this condition visible here?

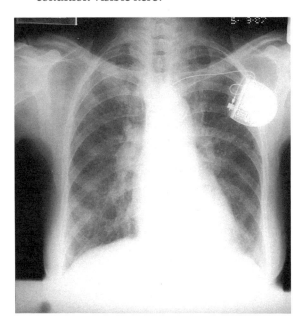

1.6
This is a colonoscopic view of a patient with bloody diarrhoea.
a) What is the abnormality?
b) What treatment would you prescribe?

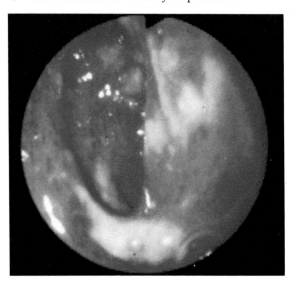

1.7
This rash developed in a patient receiving chemotherapy for Hodgkin's disease.
a) What is the diagnosis?
b) What treatment would you prescribe?

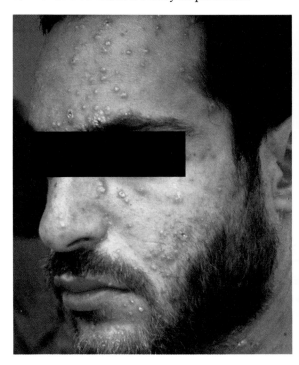

1.8
This patient also suffered from a painful knee. Give four differential diagnoses.

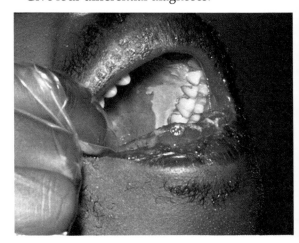

1.9

a) Describe the histological appearance.

b) Give three possible causes.

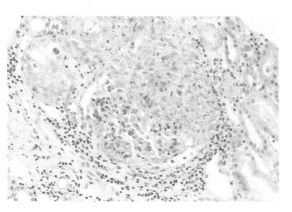

1.10

This is a CT scan of the abdomen of a traveller from Brazil who presented with jaundice, fever and abdominal pain.

a) What is the abnormality?

b) What is the likely radiological diagnosis?

c) Name two treatments.

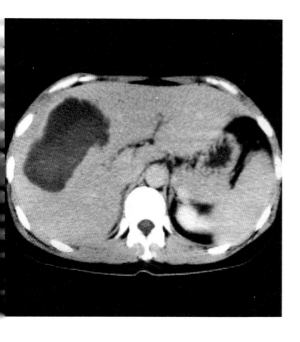

1.11

a) What is this lesion?

b) What is its likely cause?

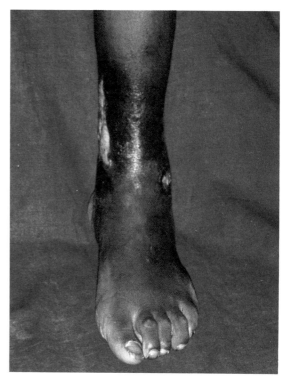

1.12

This patient complained of arthralgia and excessive post-prandial fullness.

What is the likely diagnosis?

1.13
What is the diagnosis?

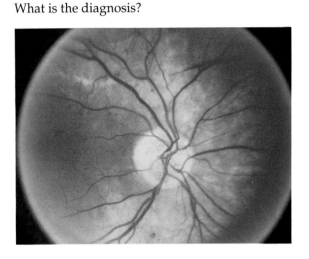

1.14
What is the diagnosis?

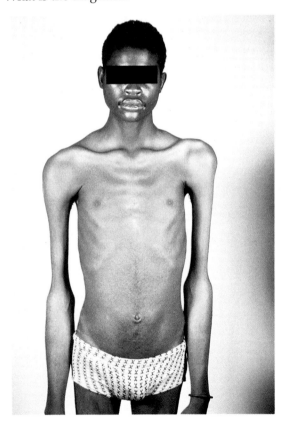

1.15
This is the peripheral blood film of a 69-year-old man who presented with herpes zoster. His blood count revealed a WBC of $70 \times 10^9/1$.
What is the diagnosis?

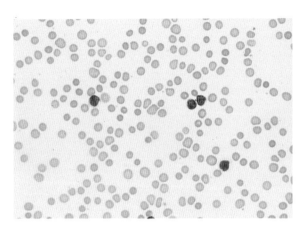

1.16
This bone marrow is taken from a patient with a pyrexia of unknown origin and hepatomegaly
a)   What is the diagnosis?
b)   Name one drug used in treatment.
c)   List one mode of transmission.

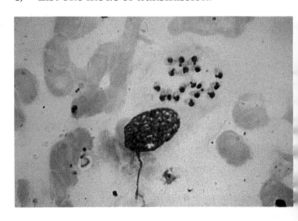

1.17

a) What is the diagnosis?

b) Name two tests you would perform to confirm your diagnosis.

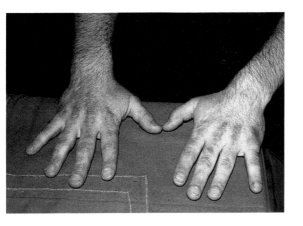

1.19

This patient is ataxic.

a) What is the diagnosis?

b) What is the mode of inheritance?

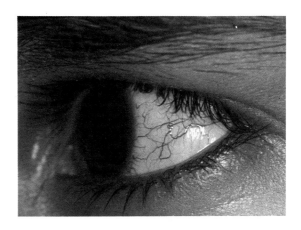

1.18

What is this physical sign?

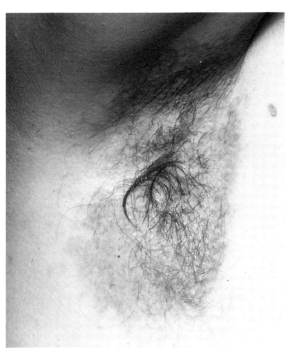

1.20

This is the peripheral blood film of a 63-year-old man with a peptic ulcer.

Suggest two haematological diagnoses.

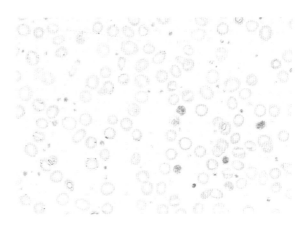

Pictorial Material Paper 2

2.1
What is the diagnosis?

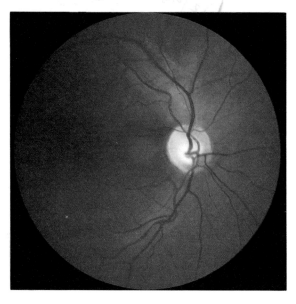

2.2
A 16-year-old boy has anaemia and splenomegaly. This is his peripheral blood film stained with brilliant cresyl blue.

What is the diagnosis?

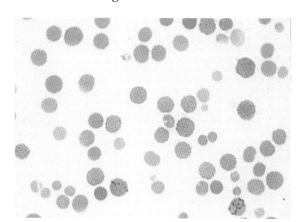

2.3
This is the chest X-ray of a patient complaining of weakness. What is the diagnosis and why is she weak?

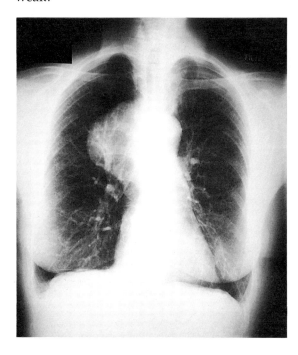

2.4
What is the diagnosis?

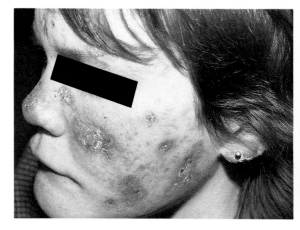

2.5
a)   What is the diagnosis?
b)   How would you treat this patient?

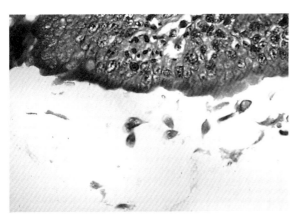

2.7
What is the abnormality?

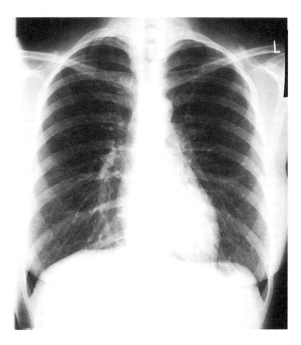

2.6
What is the diagnosis?

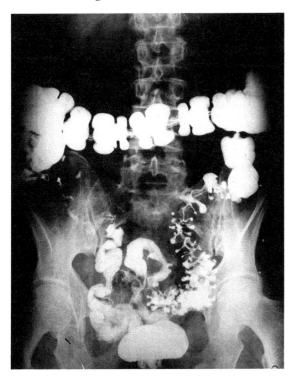

2.8
What is the diagnosis of this isolated skin lesion?

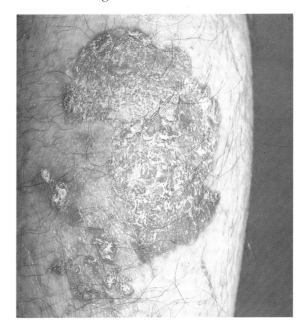

2.9

What is the diagnosis and what complication do you think has arisen?

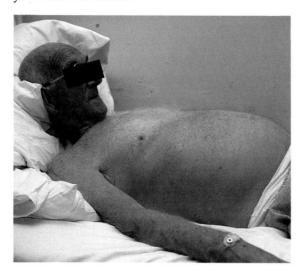

2.10

This is the peripheral blood film of a 4-year-old boy who has presented with mucous membrane bleeding.

What is the diagnosis?

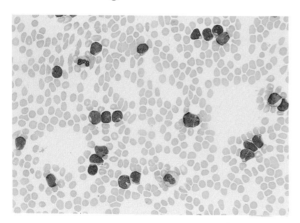

2.11

a)   What is this lesion?

b)   What is the aetiological agent?

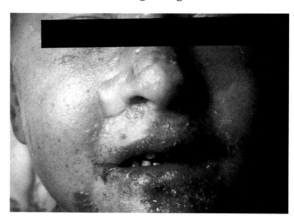

2.12

This is a barium swallow performed on a 46-year-old man.

What is the likely diagnosis?

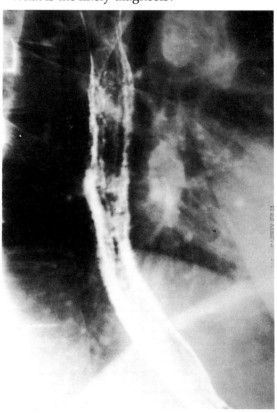

2.13
What is this condition?

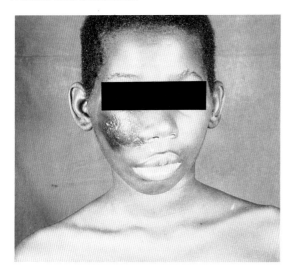

2.14
What is the diagnosis?

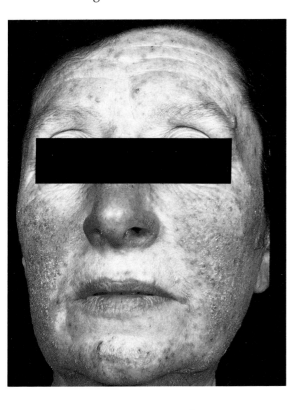

2.15
This is the peripheral blood film of a 35-year-old woman who is pale.
 What is the diagnosis?

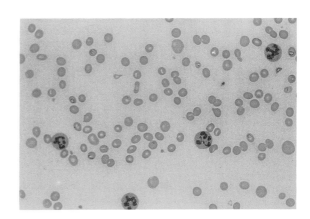

2.16
What is this lesion?

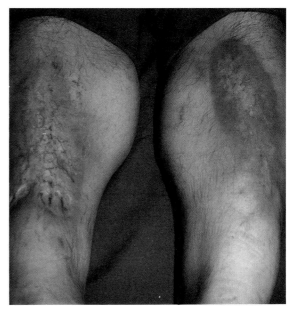

2.17

This is the plain abdominal X-ray of a 65-year-old woman with diabetes mellitus.
a)   Give two radiological abnormalities.
b)   What is the diagnosis?

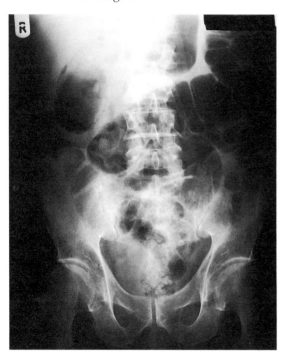

2.18

What is this scaling papular rash?

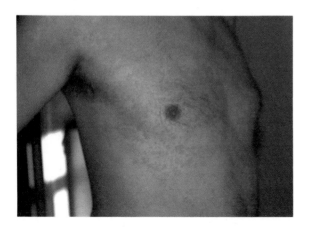

2.19

Suggest two possible diagnoses.

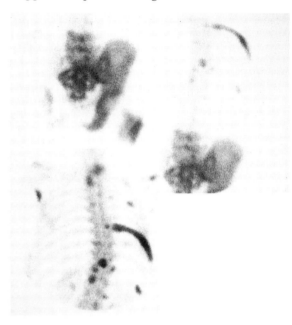

2.20

What is the most likely diagnosis in this patient with lymphadenopathy and a non-itchy rash?

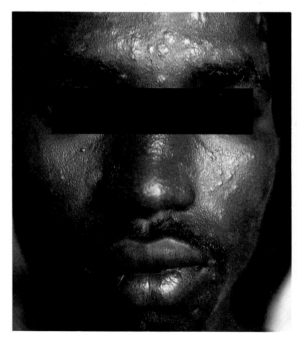

Pictorial Material Paper 3

3.1
a) What is the physical sign illustrated here?
b) What is the diagnosis?

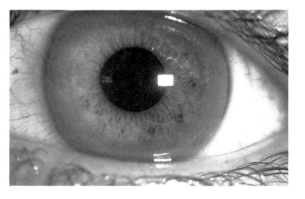

3.2
This patient also has coryza. His 5-year-old brother had a similar illness two weeks ago.
a) What is the diagnosis?
b) List two other features associated with this condition.

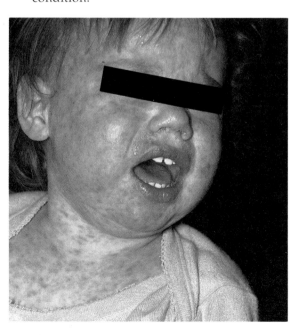

3.3
What is the likely diagnosis?

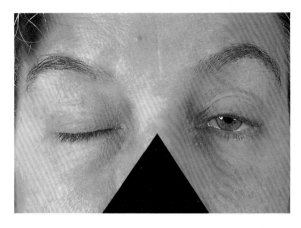

3.4
What is the diagnosis?

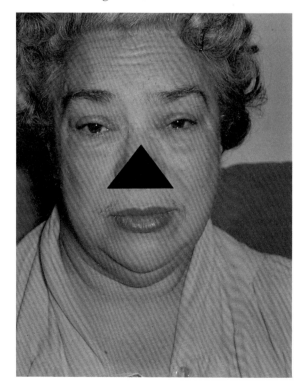

3.5
What is the diagnosis?

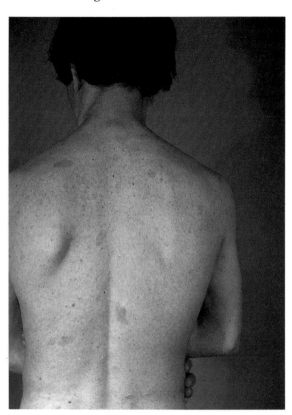

3.6
This is the peripheral blood film of a 12-year-old
girl with anaemia.
   What is the diagnosis?

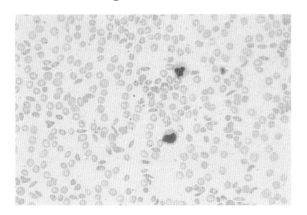

3.7
This patient had a sore throat and fever.
a)   List two abnormal physical signs.
b)   What two tests would you request to make a
     diagnosis?

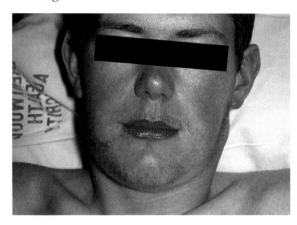

3.8
This is the intravenous urogram of a 32-year-old
man with recurrent urinary tract infections.
   What is the abnormality?

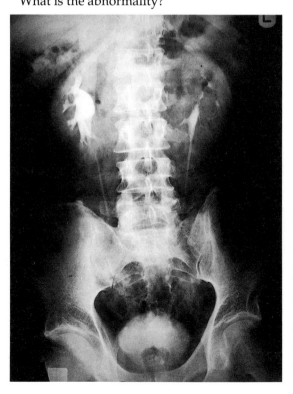

3.9

What is the diagnosis?

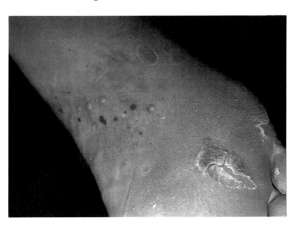

3.10

a)   What is the abnormality?

b)   What is the likely diagnosis?

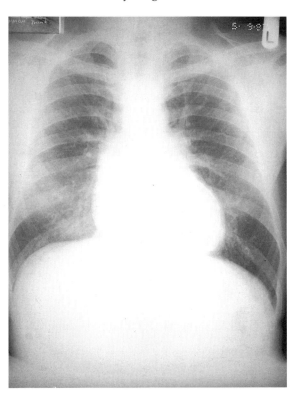

3.11

This post-mortem specimen shows a section of ileum from a patient who died after an acute febrile illness.

a)   What is the leison?

b)   What was the post-mortem diagnosis?

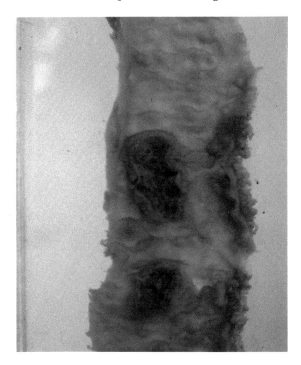

3.12

This patient was born with normal sized fingers. What is the likely diagnosis?

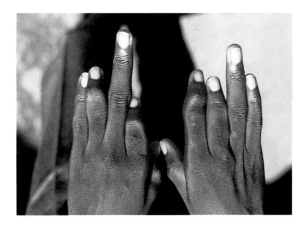

3.13
What is the diagnosis?

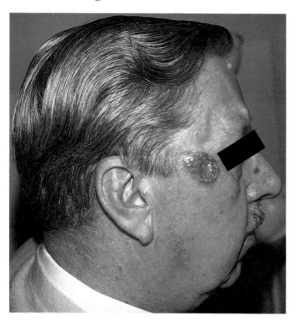

3.14
What abnormality does this MRI scan show in a previously well patient who suddenly became obtunded?

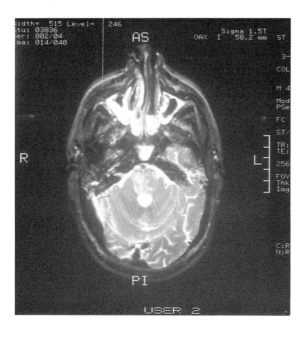

3.15
a)   What is the abnormality?
b)   Name three possible causes?

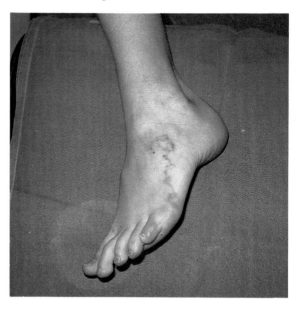

3.16
This is the peripheral blood film of a 72-year-old man with splenomegaly and anaemia.
a)   Name two abnormalities present on the film.
b)   What is the diagnosis?

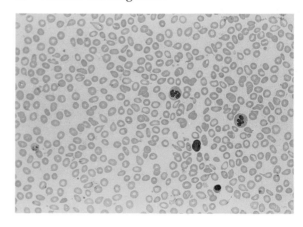

3.17
This is a barium meal of a patient who complained
of dysphagia.
   What is the diagnosis?

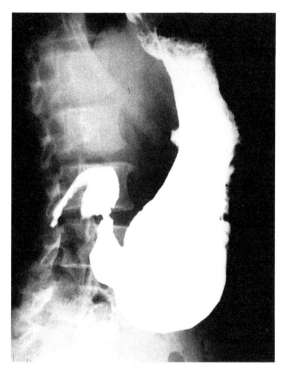

3.18
This is the blood film of a patient returning to
Britain with fever and cervical lymphadenopathy
after a 6-week holiday in East Africa.
a)   What is the diagnosis?
b)   How is this organism transmitted?

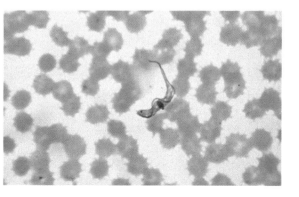

3.19
What is the diagnosis?

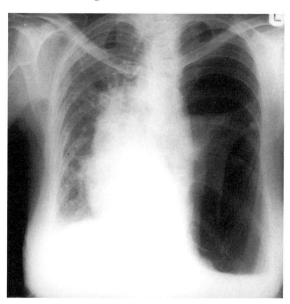

3.20
This is the peripheral blood film of a 30-year-old
man with lymphadenopathy.
   What is the diagnosis?

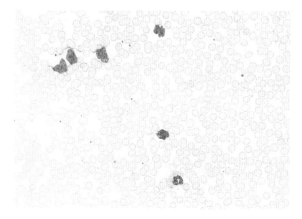

Pictorial Material Paper 4

4.1
What is the diagnosis?

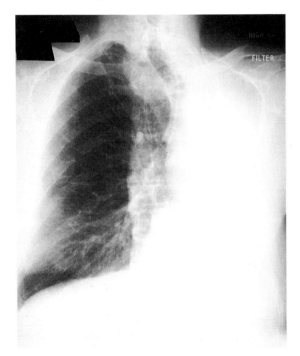

4.2
This is the blood film of a 20-year-old male with mild anaemia.

What is the diagnosis?

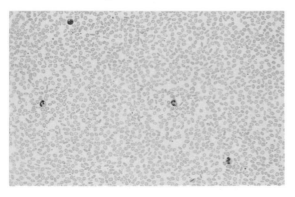

4.3
a)   What is the physical sign?
b)   What is the diagnosis?

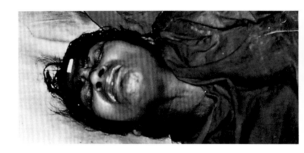

4.4
What two abnormalities are shown?

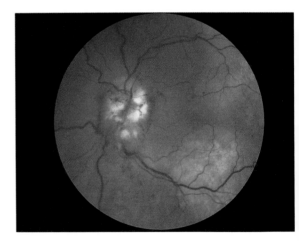

4.5
What are these lesions?

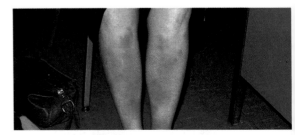

4.6

A Ziehl-Neelsen stain of a stool sample from a patient with chronic diarrhoea.
a) What is the diagnosis?
b) What one other test would you request?

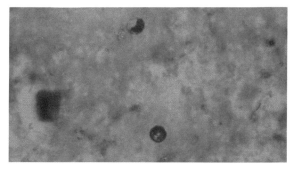

4.7

What is the diagnosis?

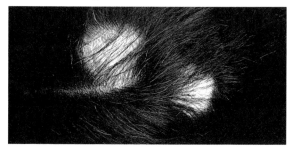

4.8

a) What is the diagnosis?
b) What is the aetiological agent?

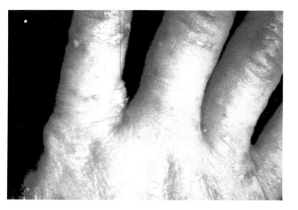

4.9

This patient also had several hypopigmented skin lesions.
a) What is the abnormality?
b) What is the diagnosis?

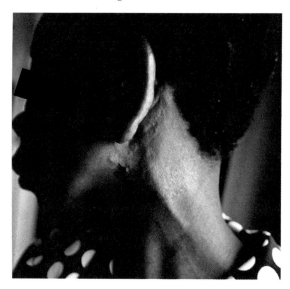

4.10

Give two diagnoses.

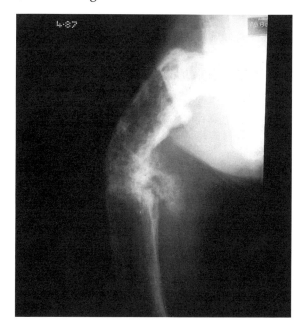

4.11

This is the peripheral blood film of a 53-year-old woman with purpura of the lower limbs.
   What is the diagnosis?

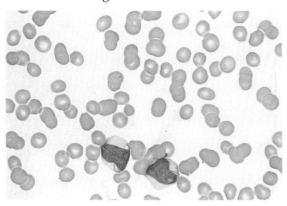

4.12

This lesion, caused by a bacterial infection, developed in a sheep farmer.
a)   What is the diagnosis?
b)   What treatment would you give?

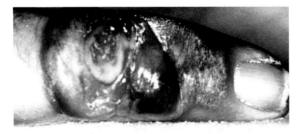

4.13

a)   List two abnormal signs.
b)   What is the diagnosis?

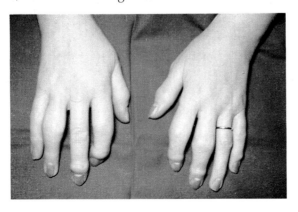

4.14

What is the abnormality?

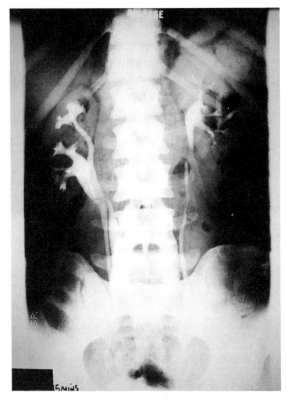

4.15

A cleaner presented to the rheumatological clinic complaining of a burning sensation in her left hand. She was referred for this investigation with diagnosis of cervical spondylosis
a)   What is the full radiological diagnosis?
b)   What is the investigation?

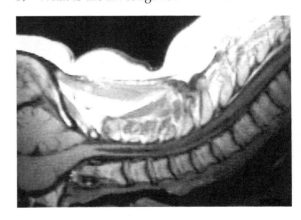

4.16
This is the peripheral blood film of an acutely unwell boy 2 weeks following a diarrhoeal illness. What is the likely diagnosis?

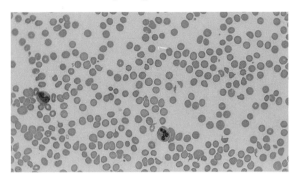

4.17
What is this lesion?

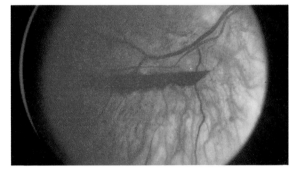

4.18
This is a section from a skin biopsy of a chronic ulcerating lesion on the side of the nose.
a) What is the pathology shown?
b) List one diagnostic possibility.

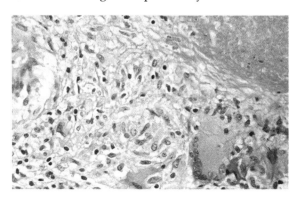

4.19
What abnormality does this ultrasound scan of the abdomen show?

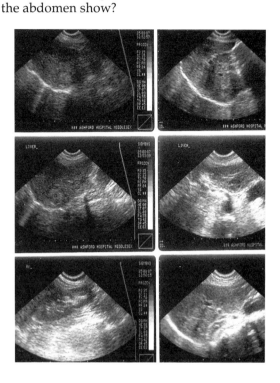

4.20
a) List four abnormalities.
b) What is the diagnosis?

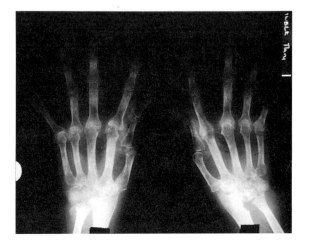

Pictorial Material Paper 5

5.1
This is the peripheral blood film of a 72-year-old man who has become anaemic.
  What is the likely diagnosis?

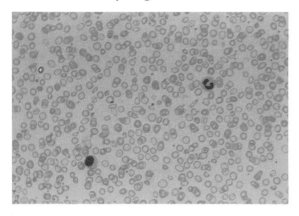

5.2
What is this skin lesion?

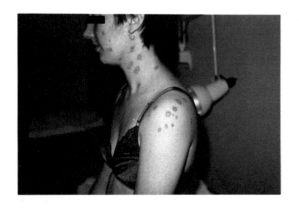

5.3
What is the abnormality?

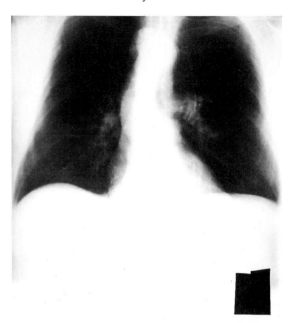

5.4
What is the abnormality?

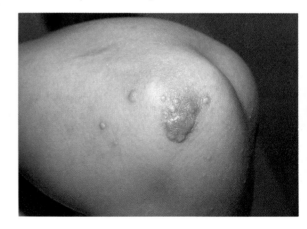

5.5
This the blood film of a 50-year-old woman with anaemia and splenomegaly.
What is the diagnosis?

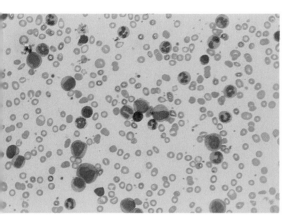

5.6
This patient was recently diagnosed as having epilepsy. He was noted to have eosinophilia a month prior to admission.
a) What is the abnormality?
b) What is the diagnosis?

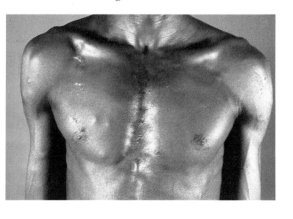

5.7
This patient had a positive faecal occult blood test.
a) What is the diagnosis?
b) List two complications.
c) What is the mode of inheritance?

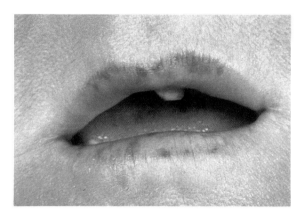

5.8
Give two abnormalities.

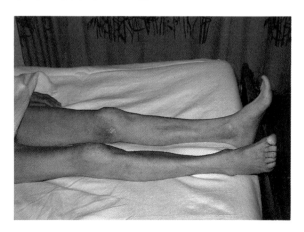

5.9
What is the diagnosis?

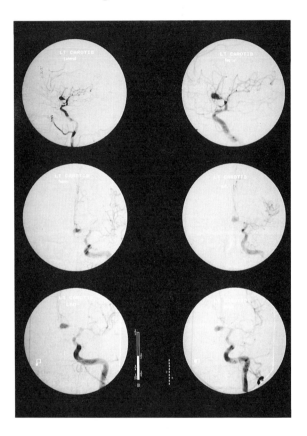

5.10
This patient returned from a safari in Kenya and complained of fever and a generalized skin rash.
a) What is the lesion?
b) List two differential diagnoses.

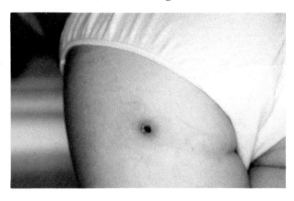

5.11
This patient complained of breathlessness.
a) Give two abnormal physical signs.
b) What is the most likely diagnosis?

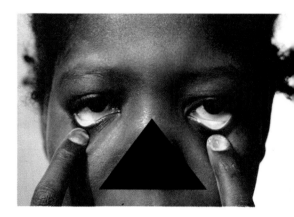

5.12
What is the diagnosis?

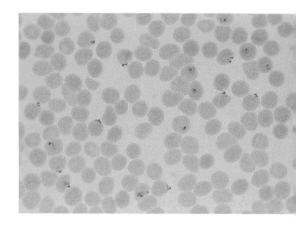

5.13

This patient had a positive faecal occult blood test.

a) What is the abnormality?

b) Name two possible underlying pathologies?

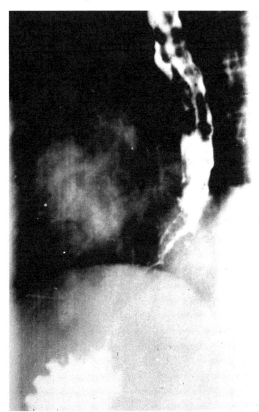

5.15

This is the peripheral blood film at 20°C of a woman who complained of recurrent abdominal pain and discolouration of her fingers following exposure to the cold.

a) What is the abnormality shown on the film?

b) What is the cause of this abnormality?

c) What is the diagnosis?

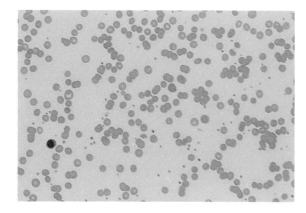

5.16

What is the diagnosis?

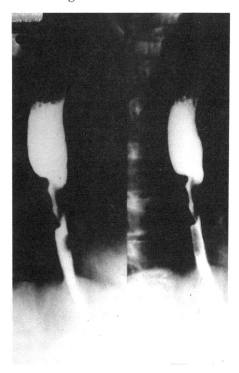

5.14

a) What is this abnormality?

b) What is the most likely underlying diagnosis?

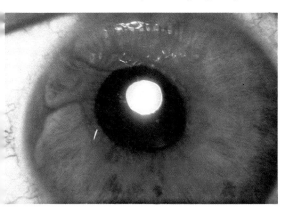

5.17

This is the bone marrow of a 49-year-old man. What is the diagnosis?

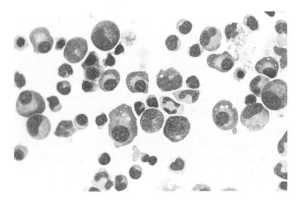

5.18

This child had a rising fever and constipation after a visit to India.
a) What physical sign is illustrated?
b) Name two investigations to confirm your diagnosis.

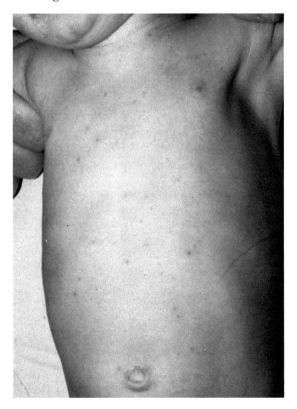

5.19

a) Name the radiological abnormalily.
b) What is the diagnosis?

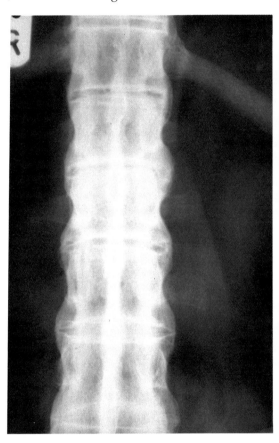

5.20

Name two abnormalities present in this fundus.

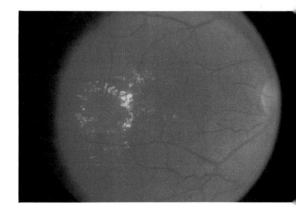

Answers to Pictorial Material Paper 1

1.1

Accepted answers

Rejected answers

Three of the following:
(a) Chemosis
Ophthalmoplegia
Exophthalmos/proptosis/lid retraction
Widening of the palpebral fissure

(b) Graves' disease

Hyperthyroidism
Thyrotoxicosis

The classic face of the patient with Graves' disease should be instantly recognisable. The condition, which has an autoimmune basis, most often affects women in their third or fourth decades. Although the eye signs are predominant, do not forget to look at the neck if it is visible – is there a goitre or a thyroidectomy scar? Other photographic features which may occur in Graves' disease include pretibial myxoedema, vitiligo (occasionally hyperpigmentation), alopecia, onycholysis, palmar erythema and spider naevi.

Note that it is not possible from this photograph to say whether the patient is hyperthyroid, euthyroid or hypothyroid. There may be other clues which might suggest thyroid status, such as 'this is a 43 year old woman with a tachycardia' in the question, but in general be careful about overinterpretation. Although in a clinical examination one only diagnoses exophthalmos or proptosis after examining the eyes from over the forehead (without which the most one can say is that the patient has lid retraction), in the written paper it is acceptable to make such a likely assumption.

1.2

Accepted answer

Acromegaly

The hands are classically 'spade like'. Everything about them is big. Relative to their length, the circumference of the fingers is particularly large.

1.3

Accepted answer

Rejected answers

Lichen planus

Psoriasis
Eczema

This purple papular lesion appears to be made up of numerous coalescing small lesions. Not visible here, a close-up would show arborizing white lines (Wickham's striae) on the surface of the lesions. Scratch marks are often also seen because it is very itchy.

1.4

Accepted answers

(a) Acanthocytes

(b) Abetalipoproteinaemia

Abnormality	*Significance*
Acanthocytes	Occur in genetic disorders of lipid metabolism
Anisocytosis	Simply means variation in size
Basophilic stippling	Represents RNA and reflects defective haemoglobin synthesis Seen in the dyserythropoietic anaemias, such as lead poisoning and thalassaemia
Burr cells	Irregularly shaped cells which occur in uraemia
Elliptocytes	Ovoid cells which occur in abundance in hereditary elliptocytosis
Howell–Jolly bodies	Nuclear remnants seen most often following splenectomy
Hypochromia	Pale-staining because of defective haemoglobinization; usually due to iron deficiency or defective haemoglobin synthesis (thalassaemia, sideroblastic anaemia)
Microcytosis	Small cells due to defective haemoglobinization. In iron deficiency, the lack of haemoglobin in the developing cell leads to an extra cell division, the result being smaller mature cells
Macrocytosis	Large cells due to dyserythropoiesis or premature release May indicate a megaloblastic anaemia (low vitamin B_{12} or folate – look for hypersegmented polymorphs) when there is one less cell division during red blood cell division Causes of simple macrocytosis include alcohol, liver disease, myelosuppressive drugs, reticulocytosis and myxoedema
Poikilocytosis	Variable shaped cells (this general description includes Burr cells, tear-drops and schistocytes)
Polychromasia	Also called anisochromasia Variation in haemoglobinization or presence in film of red blood cells of different ages (e.g. in response to bleeding, haemolysis or dyserythropoiesis)
Reticulocytes	Young, often large, red cells Signify active erythropoiesis (e.g. in haemolysis)
Schistocytes	Fragmented red cells Seen in intravascular haemolysis
Sickle cells	Characteristic of sickle cell disease
Spherocytes	Spherical cells Indicates damage to the cell membrane; may be genetic (hereditary spherocytosis) or acquired (following red cell damage, e.g. haemolysis)
Target cells	Red cells with central staining, a ring of pallor and a thin outer ring of staining Seen in deficient haemoglobinization (e.g. thalassaemia, liver disease iron deficiency anaemia and hyposplenism). In liver disease it is thought to be due to altered lipid components in the cell membrane
Tear-drop poikilocyte	A prominent feature of myelofibrosis

Acanthocytes are abnormal red blood cells which can be recognized by their spicules. If you see them in Membership, the likely diagnosis is abetalipoproteinaemia, although they may be seen in fewer numbers in severe liver disease and haemolytic anaemia (Zieve's syndrome).

Interpreting blood films in Membership

For many candidates (and at least one of the authors of this book), the prospect of interpreting blood films produces an acute feeling of nausea! The reason is simple – candidates have a reasonable chance of having come across most Membership cases in real life, but most physicians rarely, if ever, have to look at blood films.

Once again, a little focused pre-examination groundwork can pay dividends. First, try to remember what different red cell abnormalities look like. The differential diagnosis for each abnormality is often quite limited. Sometimes you are asked to describe the red cell abnormalities in addition to, or even instead of, providing a diagnosis. Cynics might say that if you can describe the appearance of the cell in Greek, you might stand a chance of getting the right answer! This may not be entirely correct, but there is some truth in it. For instance, remember that a description ending in **-cytosis** refers to the size of the cell whereas **-chromia** (or **-chromasia**) refers to haemoglobinization. It then does not take a genius to work out that microcytosis means small cells, elliptocytosis means elliptical cell or hypochromasia means pale-staining.

All this might sound patronisingly straightforward, but simple logic often deserts candidates in the examination room. If you are asked to describe the abnormalities in a blood film with red cells of variable shape and staining, you should be able to work out that they show poikilocytosis (variable shape, not to be confused with anisocytosis which is variable size) and polychromasia.

We have provided several examples of red cell abnormalities in questions in this book, but below is a diagrammatical representation of some of the abnormalities:

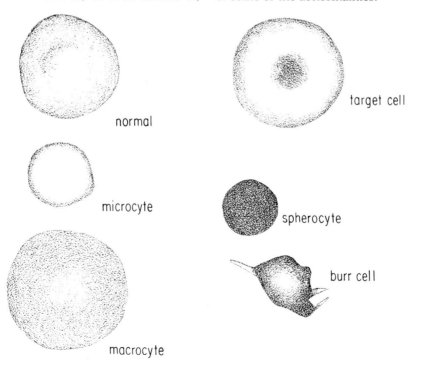

normal

microcyte

macrocyte

target cell

spherocyte

burr cell

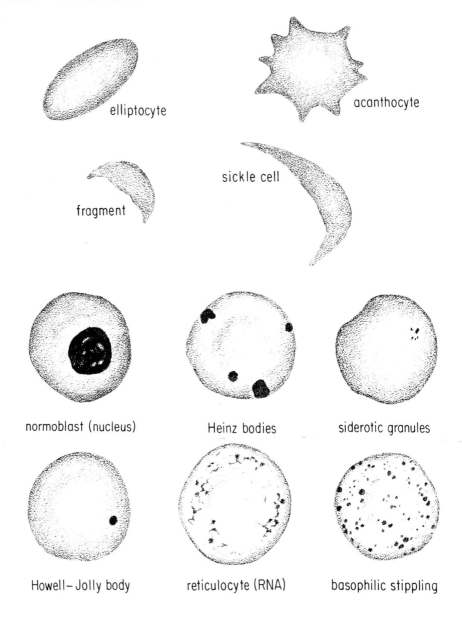

elliptocyte

acanthocyte

fragment

sickle cell

normoblast (nucleus)

Heinz bodies

siderotic granules

Howell–Jolly body

reticulocyte (RNA)

basophilic stippling

Reproduced with permission from Hoffbrand and Pettit, *Essential Haematology*; published by Blackwell Scientific Publications, 1982.

1.5

Accepted answers

(a) Sarcoidosis

(b) Reticulo-nodular shadowing in both lung fields
Pacemaker required due to heart block

Rejected answer

Pulmonary oedema due to cardiac failure

Cardiac sarcoidosis is relatively rarely a clinical problem, but heart block is the most common clinical manifestation when it occurs. An alternative diagnosis of cardiac failure causing pulmonary oedema is not really tenable because of the normal size of the heart shadow and the pattern of the pulmonary opacification.

1.6

Accepted answers

(a) Pseudomembranous colitis
Amoebic dysentery

(b) Oral vancomycin
Oral metronidazole

Rejected answers

Inflammatory bowel disease
Crohn's disease
Ulcerative colitis

The picture shows a markedly erythematous, ulcerated mucosa covered by the exudative yellow–white membrane-like material found in pseudomembranous colitis, caused by toxins A and B of *Clostridium difficile.* It usually occurs a few days after the institution of antibiotic therapy. Clindamycin, ampicillin, tetracycline, lincomycin, and the cephalosporins have been causally linked. With no clues from the history it is difficult to distinguish this from amoebic dysentery which produces similarly coloured mucosal ulceration.

The colonoscopic features of inflammatory bowel disease are usually somewhat different. Crohn's disease initially produces shallow intramucosal ulcers, but when they become as advanced as those in this picture, they are usually of bizarre shape with the surrounding mucosa forming pseudopolyps and a cobble-stone picture. In ulcerative colitis, the picture is of a granular mucosa with polyps and mucosal bridges between the ulcers.

The presence of the membrane is not essential to make a diagnosis of pseudo-membranous colitis, which can be confirmed by identifying the toxin in stool. Culture of the organism is not useful since 5% of the population carry *C. difficile.* Rectal biopsy usually demonstrates fairly characteristic changes.

Make sure the treatment you suggest is appropriate for your chosen diagnosis.

1.7

Accepted answers	*Rejected answer*
(a) Chickenpox	Shingles
(b) Intravenous acyclovir	

In an immunocompromised patient, the cause is most likely to be infective. Infective causes of papulovesicular eruptions are chickenpox, herpes simplex, smallpox, orf, and hand, foot and mouth disease. The occurrence of crops of lesions of varying ages is typical of chickenpox.

Chickenpox and shingles, in their various clinical forms, are common questions in the Membership examination. Remember to consider the systemic complications of chickenpox. For example, although relatively uncommon, acute chickenpox pneumonia is one differential diagnosis for a 'snowstorm' appearance on a chest X-ray.

1.8

Accepted answers	*Rejected answer*
Reiter's syndrome	Coeliac disease
Crohn's disease	
Ulcerative colitis	
Inflammatory bowel disease	
Behçet's syndrome	
Gonorrhoea	
HIV	

The question asks for the differential diagnosis of mouth ulceration and acute monoarthritis of a large joint. (Those of you tempted to ascribe the oral lesion to leukoplakia should have been put off by the knee pain.) Do not expect any features of the mouth ulcer itself to give any clues as to the diagnoses. It is simply a matter of going through the differential of these two features. It is particularly 'grey' because there is likely to be at least one other important clinical feature that has been omitted. While other answers are possible, these are the best and would attract highest marks.

Causes of mouth ulcers
- Idiopathic apthous ulcers
- Gastrointestinal disorders
    Crohn's disease
    Ulcerative colitis
    Coeliac disease
- Behçet's syndrome
- Reiter's syndrome
- Vasculitis
- Viral infections
    Herpes simplex
    Coxsackie
    Chickenpox
    Trigeminal zoster
    HIV
- Bacterial infections
    Secondary syphilis
    Yersinia
    Tuberculosis
    Gonorrhoea
    Vincent's angina
- Other infections
    Candida

- Primary skin disorders
    Lichen planus
    Benign mucosal pemphigoid
    Bullous pemphigoid
    Pemphigus
    Erythema bullosa
    Erythema multiforme
- Dietary deficiencies
    Iron
    Folic acid
    Vitamin B_{12} (pernicious anaemia)
    Pyridoxine
    Riboflavin
    Zinc
- Haematological disorders
    Acute leukaemia
    Neutropenia
- Malignancy
- Trauma
    False teeth
    Burns

1.9

Accepted answers

(a) Crescentic glomerulonephritis (100%)

   Rapidly progressive glomerulonephritis (50%)

(b) Systemic lupus
    Systemic vasculitis
    Goodpasture's syndrome/anti-GBM disease

> When given a gross or histological patho-
> logical specimen, first look at any
> apparently normal tissue to try and identify
> the organ you are looking at.

The apparently empty spaces around the edges of the picture could either be for air or urine. In fact, these are normal tubules – they would be very pathological pulmonary alveolar walls. Having established that this is kidney, it should become obvious that the pathological lesion in the centre of the field is a glomerulus. So what type of glomerulonephritis is this? There are three main cell types potentially involved: (a) the connective tissue cells of the supporting matrix – mesangial cells; (b) the endothelium of the glomerular capillaries; and (c) epithelium of the Bowman's capsule – the blind-ending sac of the nephron. If either or both of the first two is involved it is usually possible to make out the slim edge of the glomerulus made up of the epithelial cells. Here, the surrounding epithelial cells have enlarged, multiplied and encroached on the rest of the glomerulus. Since they surround the glomerulus circumferentially, epithelial lesions tend to grow in a crescentic fashion – hence crescentic glomerulonephritis. This is the best answer. Its usual clinical manifestation is as rapidly progressive glomerulonephritis, but the question asks for a histological diagnosis.

1.10

Accepted answers

(a) Low attenuation space occupying lesion in the right lobe of liver

(b) Amoebic liver abscess (100%)
Hepatic amoebiasis (100%)

Liver abscess (50%)

(c) Surgical drainage
Metronidazole
Tinadazole
Tetracycline
Diloxanide furoate

There is a single low attenuation area in the right lobe of the liver. Hepatic amoebic abscesses are usually single masses in the right lobe containing anchovy sauce-like material. The clinical picture is usually of swinging fever, abdominal pain and leucocytosis. Diagnosis is suggested by ultrasound, CT appearances and positive serology. Surgical drainage may be required in some cases not responsive to metronidazole or impending rupture. Diloxanide furoate is given together with metronidazole to clear the colonic cysts.

Most other causes of solitary hepatic lesions (including hydatid cysts) are unlikely to have such uniform attenuation pattern on CT. The fever suggests an infective cause, but the foreign travel favours amoebiasis over a pyogenic abscess.

Causes of space-occupying liver lesions
- Abscesses
  Amoebic
  Pyogenic
  Infected cysts/tumours
- Cysts
  Hydatid
  Congenital
- Tumours
  Primary malignant (hepatoma)
  Secondaries

1.11

Accepted answers

(a) Leg ulcer

(b) Sickle cell anaemia/disease (100%)
Tropical ulcer (100%)

Ischaemic ulcer associated with haemolytic anaemia (50%)

Rejected answers

Venous ulceration
Cellulitis
Leishmaniasis

This is a pattern recognition question. It is obvious that there is an ulcer in a young black patient. From its position and nature of the base and edges it is unlikely to be due to leishmaniasis, venous stasis, necrobiosis, pyoderma, syphilis or Wegener's granulomatosis. That leaves ischaemia due to degenerative vascular disease (unusual in this age group) or haemolytic anaemia, of which sickle cell disease would be the most common.

An alternative diagnosis would be tropical ulcer. This is a chronic necrotizing lesion which can erode down to bone. Also known as phagedaenic ulcer, it contains a mixed flora including *Borrelia vincenti* and fusiforms.

Causes of leg ulcers
Varicose veins
Ischaemic
Necrobiosis lipoidica diabeticorum
Pyoderma gangrenosum
Haemolytic anaemia
    Sickle cell anaemia
    Hereditary spherocytosis
Syphilitic
Leishmaniasis
Vasculitis (e.g. Wegener's granulomatosis)

1.12

Accepted answers

Scleroderma
Systemic sclerosis

Classical pictures of the scleroderma hand demonstrate sclerodactyly with loss of finger pulp and ulceration. This view emphasises the inflammatory component of the disease with periungual inflammation and oedema and loss of the distal interphalangeal skin folds. Raynaud's phenomenon associated with other connective tissue disorders may give this appearance, but the gastrointestinal immotility and severity of digital involvement suggest scleroderma.

1.13

Accepted answers

Proliferative diabetic retinopathy with neo-vascularization and haemorrhage affecting the optic disc (100%)

Proliferative diabetic retinopathy (50%)
Neovascularization affecting the optic disc (50%)

Diabetic retinopathy (25%)
Neovascularization (25%)

Pack as much information into your answer as possible. But don't stick your neck out too far.

Diabetic eye disease
There are three classes of changes to the eye in diabetes mellitus:
- Cataracts (six times as common as in an age-matched non-diabetic population)
- Rubeosis iridis, with its complications such as secondary glaucoma
- Retinopathy
    - (1) Background ('simple') retinopathy
        Microaneurysms or dot haemorrhages
        Hard exudates (acuity normal)
    - (2) Maculopathy (macular exudative retinopathy)
        Hard exudates and oedema near macula (acuity impaired)
    - (3) Pre-proliferative retinopathy
        Cotton wool spots
        Flame and blot haemorrhages
        Tortuous arteries
        Irregular calibre veins (indication for pan-peripheral photocoagulation of the retina)
    - (4) Proliferative retinopathy
        New vessels
        Pre-retinal/vitreous haemorrhage (e.g. subhyaloid)
        Fibrous overgrown/retinitis proliferans
        Retinal detachment

1.14

Accepted answer

Facioscapulohumeral dystrophy

Rejected answers

Marfan's syndrome
Syringomyelia

Pattern recognition again. The bilateral symmetrical wasting of the facial and shoulder muscles is striking in this patient.

> You are used to seeing neurological and degenerative disease in Caucasians and tropical diseases in Africans. Do not be put off by your colour prejudices.

1.15

Accepted answer

Chronic lymphocytic leukaemia (100%)

CLL (75%)

> Avoid abbreviations.

The high white cell count suggests a leukaemia. The blood film shows an excess of small, mature lymphocytes. The likely diagnosis is therefore CLL.

1.16

Accepted answers   *Rejected answers*

(a) Leishmaniasis (kala-azar)

(b) Pentostam/sodium stibogluconate   Mel B
    Pentamidine   Praziquantel
    Amphotericin   Tryparsamide

(c) Bite of sandfly
    Bite of *Phlebotomus/Lutzomyia* species
    Blood transfusion
    Congenital

These are Leishman–Donovan bodies (amastigotes of *Leishmania donovani*) which can be seen intra- and extracellularly. The amastigotes are ovoid with a large nucleus. The tachyzooites or bradyzooites of *Toxoplasma gondii* have a similar appearance (slightly more elongated than ovoid) but the biopsy material is usually from a fetus or cyst biopsy. If all else fails, go through a list of parasitic causes of hepatomegaly, and having excluded malaria (a purely intracellular parasite, which there is no excuse for missing), leishmaniasis should be your next choice.

1.17

Accepted answers

(a) Dematomyositis

(b) Serum creatinine phosphokinase
    Muscle biopsy
    Electromyogram

This purplish-red rash appears on the face, forehead, neck, shoulders, arms and chest. The term 'heliotrope' rash is used to describe a lilac discolouration of the eyelids. Sometimes single red, elevated smooth or scaly lesions on the knuckles (Gottron's sign, i.e. localized vasculitis), knees, elbows and maleoli are found. Redness occurs at the nail folds base and finger pads become shiny, red, atrophic and flaky. Calcinosis may occur. In adults there is 20–40% association with internal malignancy.

1.18

Accepted answer

Acanthosis nigricans

Using the 'unusual sites' approach (following), what condition involves pigmentation of the axilla? This question should trigger the answer acanthosis nigricans which typically occurs in the axillae or groin (but also may occur around the anus and involve mucous membranes). In addition to pigmentation, the skin becomes thickened with associated skin tags and warts.

The condition may be benign in the young, but in older patients it is often associated with underlying carcinoma. If all else fails, and nothing springs to mind, then the use of a 'surgical sieve', providing headings of types of pathology, might lead you to an answer.

> **The 'unusual sites' approach**
> Do not panic when shown an unusual part of the body – it is likely to be to your advantage. If nothing is obvious, ask yourself three questions:
> (1) Is there anything specific for this site that I should look for (e.g. ochronosis in the cartilage of the pinna)?
> (2) Are there any generalized lesions that are just as likely to affect this site as anywhere (e.g. Paget's disease)?
>
> If you are still stuck:
> (3) Systematically go through your 'surgical sieve' for types of pathology. Do any apply here?

> **A surgical sieve**
> Everyone, even physicians, need a 'surgical sieve': a list of headings of types of diseases to run through if your clinical creativity is on holiday. Here is one:
>
> ● Trauma or toxins
> ● Infection
> ● Neoplasm
> ● Collagen vascular/autoimmune disease
> ● Arterial/vascular disease
> ● Neurological disease
> ● Blood disease
> ● Endocrine disease
> ● Degenerative disease or drugs
> ● Stones
>
> It has the meaningless, but mercifully inoffensive, acronym of TIN CAN BEDS. It is good for non-organ specific problems, even if they present in an apparently organ-specific way, but it would miss many organ-specific conditions (e.g. asthma).

1.19

Accepted answers

(a) Ataxia telangiectasia

(b) Autosomal recessive

Rejected answers

Conjunctivitis
Wilson's disease

The picture shows telangiectasia in the eye. The question gives you the other half of the answer. Ataxia telangiectasia (AT) is an autosomal recessive disorder associated with selective IgA deficiency, cerebellar ataxia and oculocutaneous telangiectasia.

Telangiectasia of the conjunctiva may be prominent from a very early age which makes it a very useful feature for distinguishing AT from other causes of ataxia. Telangiectasia occur all over the body, not just in sun-exposed sites.

1.20

Accepted answers

Iron deficiency anaemia
Essential thrombocythaemia

Rejected answers

Hypochromasia
Microcytosis
Giant platelets

The red cells show microcytosis and hypo-chromasia characteristic of an iron deficiency anaemia. In addition, there is an abundance of platelets with several giant platelets. This suggests that the underlying cause of the peptic ulcer is essential thrombocythaemia.

Causes of a microcytic anaemia are discussed in the answer to Data Interpretation question 4.3.

Note that you are asked for diagnoses, not simply to describe the abnormalities in the film.

Answers to Pictorial Material Paper 2

2.1

Accepted answer

Optic atrophy in a negroid fundus

There should not be much difficulty with this. The danger is in overdiagnosing optic atrophy, so ensure you have looked thoroughly around the field and excluded other pathology. In this case, there is none.

2.2

Accepted answers

Haemoglobin H disease
α-Thalassaemia

Haemoglobin H is a tetramer of normal haemoglobin β-chains. It occurs when there is marked reduction in α-chain synthesis, most commonly when an individual inherits α^0-thalassaemia from one parent and α^+-thalassaemia from the other. Affected patients may survive to adult life and have less severe bone changes or growth retardation than patients with homozygous β-thalassaemia. The degrees of anaemia and splenomegaly are variable.

The numerous inclusion bodies which make the red cells look like golf balls are generated by the precipitation of Hb H under the redox action of the dye. Note also several reticulocytes; individuals usually have a haemoglobin of 7–10 g/dl and a moderate reticulocytosis.

2.3

Accepted answers

Thymic tumour
Thymoma
Myasthenia gravis

Myasthenia gravis occurs in about 30% of patients with thymic tumours. Strictly speaking, two views are required to localize a mass to a mediastinal compartment, but the answer here is in the history.

Mediastinal masses on chest X-ray
- Lymph nodes (lymphoma, metastases, granulomas, etc.)
- Thymic tumours and cysts
- Neural tumours
- Mediastinal goitres
- Teratomas
- Pericardial or pleuropericardial cysts
- Foregut duplication or cysts
- Meningocoeles
- Mediastinal abscesses
- Hiatus hernias
- Aortic aneurysms

2.4

Accepted answers

Discoid lupus erythematosus (100%)

DLE (75%)

(Systemic) lupus erythematosus (25%)
SLE (25%)

Chronic cutaneous sarcoidosis (10%)
Lupus vulgaris (10%)

As with the classical acute erythematous butterfly rash of SLE, the chronic scarring discoid lesions tend to appear in the malar region, although other sites may be affected. Discoid lesions progress from erythema and oedema to follicular plugging and telangectasia, and then atrophy with scarring and alteration in pigmentation. They usually have well-defined margins. Discoid lesions are found in about one-fifth of patients with SLE, but only 10% of patients with chronic discoid lesions go on to develop any other feature of lupus. This lesion is rather distinctive clinically. Unusually, sarcoidosis, tuberculosis or lichen planus could produce a similar pattern.

2.5

Accepted answers

(a) Giardiasis

(b) Metronidazole
    Tinidazole

Rejected answers

Coeliac disease
Tropical sprue

This picture shows a jejunal biopsy specimen with villous atrophy due to giardiasis. The organism is seen in the lumen. *Giardia lamblia* is a flagellated protozoan which colonizes and multiplies within the small intestine, often without detriment to the host. The trophozoite is ovoid in shape and contains a central axostyle (rod) and two sucking discs which appear as 'eyes' and give it its characteristic appearance. Symptoms such as anorexia, nausea, borborygmi, dyspepsia and diarrhoea may occur. Malabsorption and steatorrhoea may occur and are thought to be due to damage to villi. This ranges from mild changes such as partial villous atrophy to total villous atrophy. Cysts and trophozoites may be found in the stool but a negative examination does not exclude the diagnosis. Jejunal aspirates may increase diagnostic yield. Metronidazole or tinidazole are treatments of choice. Mepacrine can also be used but has a lower cure rate. Tinidazole has the advantage of requiring only a single dose.

2.6

Accepted answer

Diverticular disease

Rejected answers

Diverticulitis
Multiple polyposis

Diverticula are frequently found in the colon in 50% of patients over the age of 50 years. Diverticulitis is inflammation of these diverticula. Diverticular disease is asymptomatic in 90% of cases. In the rest it may present as constipation, pain in the left iliac fossa and frequent passage of loose stools. Diagnosis is made on barium enema, as in this case.

Complications of diverticular disease
- Diverticulitis
    - Abscess formation
    - Perforation
    - Fistula formation
    - Intestinal obstruction
- Rectal bleeding
- Iron deficiency anaemia

Diagnoses often missed on barium enemas
- Pneumatosis cystoides intestinalis
    - Multiple gas-filled cysts in the submucosa of the colon
- Ischaemic colitis
    - 'Thumb printing' and strictures
- Polyps
    - Solitary polyp
    - Familial colonic polyposis
    - Gardener's syndrome
- Intussusception
    - Ileo-caecal
- Normal barium enema but incidental finding of
    - Bamboo spine
    - Pancreatic calcification
    - Dense vertebra
- Silhouette of *Ascaris lumbricoides*

2.7

Accepted answers

Right cervical rib (100%)

Cervical rib (75%)

Places to look on the chest X-ray for subtle abnormalities
- Behind the heart (?prosthetic valves, increased densities, air shadows)
- Hilar regions (?left higher than right as is normal, ?symmetrical density)
- Costophrenic angles
- Look along both diaphragms and up the sides of the lungs (?calcification, pleural plaques)
- Mediastinum, particularly scrutinize the region of clavicles and suprasternal notch (?tracheal compression, ?retrosternal goitre, erosions of the medial ends of the clavicles)
- Lung apices
- Bones of the thoracic cage (?fracture, rib-notching, ribs missing, cervical ribs)
- Breast shadows
- Check both arms are present!
- Any abnormality below diaphragm

The difficulty in this question is simply spotting the abnormality.

When an immediate diagnosis is not apparent, develop a systematic routine for examining the projected material, whether it be a chest X-ray, a pair of hands or a face.

What is important is not that you follow a particular routine, but that you devise one in the first place – and learn to stick to it. We offer one such routine for examining chest X-rays.

2.8

Accepted answer

Bowen's disease of the skin

Rejected answers

Mycosis fungoides
Psoriasis

Usually a single well-defined lesion, red scaly and often slightly pigmented, it looks not unlike a single patch of psoriasis. A third of patients have multiple lesions. In non-exposed areas, think of underlying arsenic poisoning.

> If you think you are being shown a single patch of psoriasis, ask: could it be Bowen's disease?

2.9

Accepted answers

Haemochromatosis with ascites (100%)

Cirrhosis with ascites (50%)

The most striking feature is this man's ascites. Are there any clues as to the cause? His face shows marked pigmentation. Hence the link. The pigmentation is not jaundice, otherwise any cause of cirrhosis could explain the picture.

> If you cannot see anything unusual in a slide, go back and ask yourself about generalized disorders of pigmentation. They are easy to miss.

2.10

Accepted answers

Acute lymphoblastic leukaemia (100%)

ALL (75%)

Acute leukaemia (10%)

In Membership, the combination of this history and a blood film is suggestive of acute leukaemia! This is confirmed by the film which shows an excess of undifferentiated blast cells. The difficulty usually lies in discriminating between acute myeloid and acute lymphocytic leukaemias. Here the cells are morphologically lymphocytes and the age is right for ALL.

2.11

Accepted answers

(a) Impetigo

(b) *Staphylococcus aureus*
Group A *Streptococcus*
β-Haemolytic *Streptococcus*

Typically, the facial skin is affected with crusting and bullous lesions. Impetigo is usually due to *Staphylococcus* but is sometimes due to *Streptococcus* or even a mixture of both. It comprises multiple, discrete whitish-creamish lesions. The lesions may rupture leaving a raw erythematous area with crusting.

2.12

Accepted answer

Oesophageal candidiasis

The X-ray shows fine ulceration extending throughout the oesophagus. Oesophageal candidiasis is the likely diagnosis, but a similar appearance could occur following cytomegalo-virus or herpes simplex infection.

The other causes of oesophageal candidiasis include immunosuppression of any kind (AIDS, transplant recipients, chemotherapy, etc.).

Diagnosis to look out for in barium swallows
- Oesophageal/pharyngeal pouch
- Oesophageal diverticulum
- Achalasia
- Carcinoma
- Benign stricture
- Oesophageal web
- Varices

- Oesophageal candidiasis/oesophagitis
- Hiatus hernia
- Extrinsic pressure (nodes/aneurysms/left atrium)
- May be normal with other pathology, e.g.
  Bamboo spine
  Cervical rib
  Soft tissue calcification

2.13

Accepted answer

Chloroma

This soft tissue mass of leukaemic cells, a chloroma, has greenish discolouration around a bruise-like lesion. This is the only patho-gnomic lesion of any of the leukaemias, named for its green colour (which is due to myelo-peroxidase in the cells of acute granulocytic leukaemia).

2.14

Accepted answer

Rosacea

Rejected answer

Dermatitis

This woman has diffuse facial erythema with papules and pustules. Her skin looks tense and shiny, and (although difficult to see) she has numerous telangiectasia. This is the characteristic appearance of rosacea. Thirty per cent of patients have associated keratoconjunctivitis.

2.15

Accepted answer

Megaloblastic anaemia

Rejected answers

Folate deficiency
Vitamin B_{12} deficiency

The blood film shows hypersegmented polymorphonuclear cells characteristic of megaloblastic anaemia. Although folate deficiency and vitamin B_{12} deficiency are the most common causes of this anaemia, it is not possible to ascertain the exact cause from this blood film. Thirty-five is a little young for pernicious anaemia.

2.16

Accepted answers

Necrobiosis lipoidica
Necrobiosis lipoidica diabeticorum

This characteristic lesion appears as a red-brown patch and slowly enlarges and becomes yellow and atrophic. As almost a half of these patients do not have diabetes, it is reasonable not to use the word 'diabeticorum'.

2.17

Accepted answers

(a) Air (gas) in the gall bladder and gall bladder wall
   Intestinal ileus (small bowel and large bowel)

(b) Emphysematous cholecystitis

Rejected answer

Gall stone ileus

The diagnosis here is emphysematous cholecystitis because air can be seen in the wall of the gall bladder. The condition, due to infection, most commonly occurs in elderly female diabetics and is usually caused by coliforms.

Causes of gas in the biliary tree

- Within the bile ducts
  (a) Incompetence of the sphincter of Oddi following sphincterotomy, passage of a gallstone or in the elderly ('patulous sphincter')
  (b) Post-operative cholecystectomy or choledochoenterostomy
  (c) Spontaneous biliary fistula due to passage of gallstone from gall-bladder to bowel, duodenal ulcer perforating into common bile duct, tumour or malignancy

- Within the gall-bladder
  (a) All of the above
  (b) Emphysematous cholecystitis

2.18

Accepted answer

Pityriasis versicolor

Rejected answer

Pityriasis rosea

This lesion has numerous small papules, typically on the trunk and arms with fine scaling. They may be brown, pink or de-pigmented and are especially obvious after tanning. Pityriasis rosea appears in rows roughly parallel to the ribs and you are likely to be shown a typical herald patch with it.

2.19

Accepted answers

Paget's disease of bone
Bone metastases

Radiologically, this is more likely to be Paget's disease because of the assymetrical distribution of the lesions and also their hemipelvic distribution. However, multiple sclerotic bony metastases cannot be excluded.

2.20

Accepted answer

Secondary syphilis

Primary skin diseases do not usually have associated lymphadenopathy, so the question tells you to look for a systemic disease. Of the causes for lymphadenopathy the only one likely to cause this type of lesion is syphilis in its secondary stage.

Causes of lymphadenopathy
- Inflammatory
  - Pyogenic
  - Non-pyogenic infection
  - Autoimmune disease
- Granulomatous
  - Sarcoidosis
  - Tuberculosis
  - Syphilis
  - Toxoplasmosis
  - Systemic fungal infection (e.g. histo-plasmosis)
- Malignant
  - Lymphoma
  - Leukaemia
  - Carcinoma
  - Melanoma
  - Sarcoma
- Drugs
  - Phenytoin
- Endocrine
  - Addison's disease
  - Thyrotoxicosis
- Congenital
  - Lymphangioma
  - Cystic hygroma

Answers to Pictorial Material Paper 3

3.1

Accepted answers

(a) Kayser–Fleischer ring

(b) Wilson's disease
Hepatolenticular degeneration

A rare truly pathognomonic physical sign.

3.2

Accepted answers

(a) Measles
Rubeola

(b) Cough
Koplik's spots
Conjunctivitis
Convulsions
Otitis media

Rejected answers

Rubella
Roseola infantum
Exanthem subitum

The rash of measles occurs initially on the forehead and then spreads rapidly to involve the rest of the body. At first the rash is discrete but later becomes confluent and patchy. It is dark red initially then fades in a week leaving a brownish discolouration with desquamation. In rubella a short-lived pink macular rash (if it occurs at all) starts behind the ears and on the forehead and spreads to the face, trunk and limbs. In roseola infantum (also known as exanthem subitum) the rash is pink more like rubella, than measles. The rash in this picture is typical of measles.

Viral causes of maculopapular rash	
Measles (synonym: rubeola)	Adenovirus
Rubella (synonym: German measles)	Parvovirus
Epstein–Barr virus	Enterovirus
Cytomegalovirus	Hepatitis B

3.3

Accepted answers

(a) Ocular myasthenia (100%)
Myasthenia gravis (100%)

Myasthenia (50%)

The signs here are of a right complete and left incomplete ptosis with a normal pupil. The arched eyebrows, caused by an overactive frontalis muscle, demonstrate that the patient is trying to open her eyes. A third nerve palsy does cause a complete ptosis and there is no clue as to any ophthalmoplegia of the underlying eyeball. However, the position of the left eyeball makes a complete third nerve palsy unlikely, and the normal pupil excludes a Horner's syndrome. We are left with generalized muscle diseases, of which the most likely is myasthenia. The facial muscles are the earliest to be involved. Some might prefer the term ocular myasthenia, as that is all that can be deduced from the picture. However, the condition is known as myasthenia gravis, so that is also an acceptable answer. Always think of myasthenia when presented with 'funny' ophthalmoplegias.

3.4

Accepted answers

Myxoedema
Hypothyroidism

Rejected answer

Acromegaly

The coarseness of features in hypothyroidism is sometimes mistaken for acromegaly. This lady has the puffy features and dry skin typical of hypothyroidism.

3.5

Accepted answers

Von Recklinghausen's neurofibromatosis

Although this young man does not have florid prominent neurofibromatoses, he has many café-au-lait spots. The presence of six or more in an adult, greater than 1.5 cm in diameter, is diagnostic of neurofibromatosis until proven otherwise. The other causes of multiple café-au-lait spots are too rare to be encountered in the examination.

3.6

Accepted answer

Sickle cell disease

Sickle cells can clearly be seen on the film. Note also the typical ansiochromasia and poikilocytosis.

3.7

Accepted answers

(a) Cervical lymphadenopathy
Malar flush

(b) Paul–Bunnell test
Monospot™ test
EBV IgM
CMV serology
Toxoplasma dye test
HIV test
Full blood count and differential
Throat swab
ASOT titre

Cervical lymphadenopathy, rash and sore throat can be due to several infectious agents: EBV, CMV, *Toxoplasma gondii, Streptococcus pyogenes,* and rubella. It is also a feature of Kawasaki's disease in children. The age favours EBV, but this is a question about the differential diagnosis.

3.8

Accepted answer

Horseshoe kidney

The pelvi-caliceal systems are rotated, the kidneys are closer to the mid-line than normal and a bridge of renal tissue extends across the mid-line at the lower poles. This is associated with an increased incidence of infection, renal calculi and transitional cell carcinoma.

3.9

Accepted answers

Pustular psoriasis
Keratoderma blenorrhagica
Reiter's syndrome

The cutaneous features of Reiter's syndrome affecting palms and soles, known as keratoderma blenorrhagica, resemble pustular psoriasis, with which it is anyway associated, both being linked to HLA-B27. Macules, papules, vesicles and pustules occur as do thickening, hyperkeratosis and crusting. This man actually had pustular psoriasis. Although Reiter's syndrome would pass, one would expect more inflammation.

3.10

Accepted answers

(a) Pericardial calcification

(b) Tuberculous pericarditis

Rejected answer

Left ventricular aneurysm

Either you see it or you don't!

3.11

Accepted answers

(a) Ulcers of the ileal mucosa

(b) Typhoid
    Yersinia

Rejected answers

Schistosomiasis
Carcinoid
Amoebiasis
Tuberculosis
Crohn's disease

Whilst the rule for ulcers is 'longitudinal ulcers for typhoid' and 'transverse ulcers for tuberculosis' this is not hard and fast. Small bowel ulcers can also occur in Crohn's disease.

However, typhoid or *Yersinia* remains the best answer, because neither tuberculosis nor Crohn's qualify as the acute febrile illness of the history.

3.12

Accepted answers

Sickle cell anaemia
Sickle cell disease
Juvenile chronic arthritis

Unequal fingers in a patient born with normal sized fingers in the absence of trauma is most likely due to repeated episodes of inflammation and joint destruction or to infarction. The fact that the patient is black makes the diagnosis of sickle cell anaemia more likely.

3.13

Accepted answers

Rodent ulcer
Basal cell carcinoma

This lesion has the pearly-white edge with a rolled border typical of a basal cell carcinoma (BCC). Any such lesion is to be considered a BCC until biopsy proves otherwise. Keratoacanthoma is sometimes mistaken for a BCC, but BCCs tend to ulcerate in the centre whereas keratoacanthomas, as their name suggests, produce keratin. Squamous cell carcinomas do not have this rolled pearly white margin.

3.14

Accepted answers

Pontine or brain stem haemorrhage

This depends on having two pieces of knowledge: that the dense region in the centre of the posterior fossa is pathological and that at this level it is visualizing the pons. With those two pieces of information plus the sudden onset, this is likely to be pontine haemorrhage. Central pontine myelinosis could adopt this appearance, but is excluded by the history.

3.15

Accepted answers

(a) Cutaneous larva migrans

(b) Animal hookworms:
     Ankylostoma braziliense (dog; cat)
     Ankylostoma caninum
     Uncinaria stenocephala
     Bunostomum phlebotomum
  Human hookworms:
     Necator americanum
     Ankylostoma duodenale

Rejected answers

Erythema marginatum
Scabies

Acceptable for full marks:
Any of the above genus or genus + species
Latin names
Hookworm

Cutaneous larva migrans is characterized by this serpiginous, raised, erythematous pruritic skin lession.

3.16

Accepted answers

(a) Tear-drop poikilocytes (100%)
Nucleated red cells (100%)

Anisocytosis (50%)

Poikilocytosis (25%)

(b) Myelofibrosis
Myelosclerosis

Rejected answer

Leuko-erythroblastic blood film

The blood film shows tear-drop poikilocytes which are characteristic of myelofibrosis. The presence of nucleated red cells is also characteristic of this condition. Anisocytosis also occurs, but is not very marked on this particular film. Strictly, bone marrow examination is necessary to confirm the diagnosis.

3.17

Accepted answers

Achalasia of the cardia
Achalasia of the oesophagus
Cardiospasm

Rejected answer

Carcinoma

Failure of relaxation of the lower oesophageal sphincter and of oesophageal peristalsis causes dysphagia. Solids and liquids are swallowed only slowly and stasis of food with oesophageal expansion occurs. Other pictures of achalasia that may be shown include a chest X-ray with an air/fluid level behind the heart and/or a double right heart border produced by a grossly expanded oesophagus.

3.18

Accepted answers

(a) Trypanosomiasis
African trypanosomiasis
Nagana
Trypanosoma rhodesiense infection
Trypanosoma brucei infection

(b) Tse-tse fly bite
Glossina species bite
Receipt of infected blood products

African trypanosomiasis can be caused by two morphologically indistinguishable trypanosome species: *Trypanosoma brucei rhodesiense* (East and Central Africa) or *Trypanosoma brucei gambiense* (West Africa). These are transmitted by the bite of a tse-tse fly (*Glossina* spp).

African sleeping sickness is also called by the name 'Nagana'. South American trypanosomiasis (Chagas' disease) is caused by *Trypanosoma cruzi* and is transmitted by bugs belonging to the Reduvidae family, infective faeces being rubbed into skin or conjunctiva. Since both forms can be present in the blood, contaminated blood can very rarely be a source of infection. (In the presence of complete ignorance, this would have been a good guess, with nothing to be lost.) African trypanosomiasis is distinguishable from South American by the geographical origin of the patient and by the morphological appearance of the parasite: *T. cruzi* is slightly larger, has a prominent kinetoplast at the end and is C-shaped.

Blood films and diagnosis of infection

- Malaria
    Plasmodium spp.
        P. falciparum
        P. malariae
        P. vivax
        P. ovale
- Babesiosis
    Babesia spp
- Trypanosomiasis
    Trypanosoma spp.
        T. brucei rhodesiense
        T. brucei gambiense
        T. cruzi

- Leishmaniasis
    Leishmania donovani
- Filariasis
    Wuchereria bancrofti
    Brugia malayi
    Dipetolema perstans
    Loa loa
    Mansonella ozzardi
- Borreliosis
    Borrelia recurrentis
- Bartonellosis
    Bartonella baccilliformis

3.19

Accepted answers	*Rejected answer*
Left tension pneumothorax (100%)	Left pneumothorax
Tension pneumothorax (75%)	

Despite the presence of a left pleural adhesion, there is no doubt about the diagnosis. The whole mediastinum (including the heart) has been pushed across.

3.20

Accepted answer	*Rejected answer*
Viral illness	Leukaemia

The blood film shows the abnormal ('atypical') lymphocytes (often called mononuclear cells) of a viral infection. Given the history and these cells it is impossible to distinguish infectious mononucleosis and cytomegalovirus (or, less likely, toxoplasmosis) infection. Note that the cells are more pleomorphic than leukaemic cells, with which they might be confused. The cytoplasmic enhancement seen when the lymphocyte membrane lies adjacent to red blood cells also helps to make the distinction.

Answers to Pictorial Material Paper 4

4.1

Accepted answer

Left pneumonectomy
Total collapse of the left lung

In the original X-ray surgical clips could be seen ligating the stump of the left main bronchus, indicating a previous left pneumonectomy.

4.2

Accepted answer

Hereditary elliptocytosis

The blood film shows more than 50% oval cells (elliptocytes), which should lead to the diagnosis of hereditary elliptocytosis. The presence of pencil cells and other poikilocytes in the film is typical of this condition. Note that elliptocytes can also be seen in thalassaemias and iron deficient anaemias.

4.3

Accepted answers

(a) Risus sardonicus
     Trismus

(b) Tetanus

The sardonic smile of tetanus (risus sardonicus) due to tonic muscle spasm of the facial and neck muscles is illustrated. This is evidence of end-stage of the disease and there will be considerable difficulty in swallowing and breathing capacity. Tonic muscle spasm remains between reflex convulsions and this distinguishes it from strychnine poisoning.

4.4

Accepted answers

Choroidal metastasis
Papilloedema

Choroidal metastases are the most common intraocular malignancy. They are often indistinct with minimal retinal elevation, and a mottled appearance due to overlying pigment epithelium. While often painful, vision is usually unaffected. They are often bilateral and there is usually a history of malignant disease. Treatment of choice is local radiotherapy.

Blurring of disc margins with engorged veins and haemorrhage at and around the disc are the characteristic findings of papilloedema.

4.5

Accepted answers

Erythema nodosum

These tender lesions, characteristically occurring on the shins, are a vasculitic response to a variety of insults, the most common of which are drugs (contraceptive pill, sulphonamides, penicillin), infections (strepto-coccal, mycobacterial, *Yersinia*, brucellosis and fungi), a variety of systemic disorders such as inflammatory bowel disease, sarcoidosis and Behçet's disease, and pregnancy.

4.6

Accepted answers

(a) Cryptosporidiosis
    Cryptosporidium parvum

(b) HIV test

Rejected answers

Isospora
Giardia
Mycobacteria/TB

Ziehl–Neelsen staining on stool samples is used for detection of mycobacteria or crypto-sporidia. The latter are easily identified by red staining of the ovoid or circular oocyst.

4.7

Accepted answer

Alopecia areata

The diagnosis is made by virtue of the lack of scarring, the well-demarcated patches, and the 'exclamation mark' stumps of hair around the edges of the patches.

4.8

Accepted answers

(a) Scabies

(b) *Sarcoptes scabiei*

Scabies is an allergy to the faeces of the mite *Sarcoptes scabiei*. Papules, vesicles and excoriations are seen and the most affected areas are the finger webs, axillae, nipple areolae, buttock folds, wrist flexures and penis, where it is associated with papules in nine out of ten males.

4.9

Accepted answers

(a) Thickening of greater auricular nerve

(b) Leprosy

Leprosy is the most common cause of peripheral neuropathy on a worldwide basis. It is a chronic granulomatous disease caused by *Mycobacterium leprae* and causes a spectrum of illnesses in humans. At one end of the spectrum is the high resistance form, tuberculoid leprosy, which is characterized by a few hypopigmented lesions with thickened superficial nerves. The centres of these lesions are often anaesthetic. Lepromatous leprosy is the low resistance form with extensive, bilaterally symmetrical, diffuse skin involvement. Loss of eyebrows (madurosis), leonine facies, thickened skin, nasal collapse and saddle nose, and keratitis and iridocyclitis make good examination material.

4.10

Accepted answers

Paget's disease of bone

Osteosarcoma

The femur is abnormally shaped with coarsened trabeculae and a thickened medial cortex. The radiological distinction between active and inactive disease is irrelevant for Membership purposes.

Sarcomatous change occurs in 10% of patients with widespread Paget's disease, commonly osteosarcoma of femur, humerus or pelvis. The calcified projection around a metaphysis is a characteristic appearance.

4.11

Accepted answers

Acute myeloid leukaemia

Rejected answers

Acute leukaemia

The blood film shows two blast cells each with an Auer rod in the cytoplasm. Auer rods are only seen in myeloid lineage cells and almost always in myeloblasts. In Membership, an Auer rod means AML.

4.12

Accepted answers

(a) Anthrax

(b) Penicillin

An eschar on the finger of a farmer, caused by a bacterial infection, suggests anthrax. (In the UK, the viral infection orf is a more common cause of such an eschar.) Anthrax is caused by *Bacillus anthracis* and transmission is by direct contact with an infected animal. It is seen in farmers, butchers, and wool and hide dealers. The cutaneous form is the most common presentation and is self-limiting in most cases. The lesion is typically erythematous and maculopapular, and eventually forms vesicles and ulcers with a black eschar in the centre. Diagnosis is by demonstration of organism in smears and culture and by detection of a four-fold rise in antibody titres on ELISA testing of paired sera. Penicillin is the drug of choice although chloramphenicol and tetracycline have also been used successfully.

4.13

Accepted answers

(a) Heberden's nodes
    Bouchard's nodes

(b) Osteoarthritis

These eponymous nodes are, in fact, osteophytes.

Commonly illustrated hand lesions
- Joints
    Arthritis mutilans (psoriasis)
    Rheumatoid arthritis
    Osteoarthritis (Heberden's and Bouchard's nodes)
    Gout
    Jaccoud's arthropathy (SLE)
- Fingers
    Rash over knuckles
        Dermatomyositis
        Granuloma annulare
    Thick hands of acromegaly
    Marfan's fingers
    Claw hand
    Vasculitis/digital gangrene
    Calcinosis
    Scelerodactyly
- Other
    Small muscle wasting (motor neurone disease/T1 lesion)
    Wasting of first dorsal interosseous (Pancoast's tumour)
    Vitiligo
    Psoriatic rash
    Palmar erythema
    Palmar xanthoma

4.14

Accepted answer

Partial duplex of the right kidney

This is the most common anomaly of the urinary tract and is found in about 4% of individuals. It is usually unilateral and more common on the left side than the right.

4.15

Accepted answers

(a) Syringomyelia with herniation of the cerebellar tonsils

(b) Magnetic resonance imaging of the cervical spine

The radiological diagnosis is easy, especially with the history of loss of pain sensation. The asymmetry in the history is a trick; a syrinx may expand in one direction more than the other. The tonsillar herniation, a not-infrequent association, is hinted at by the reference to a 'full' diagnosis.

4.16

Accepted answer

Haemolytic uraemic syndrome

Rejected answers

Microangiopathic haemolytic anaemia
Disseminated intravascular haemolysis

The blood film shows fragmented red cells characteristic of a microangiopathic haemolytic anaemia (MAHA). However, given the history, the likely diagnosis is the haemolytic uraemic syndrome (HUS).

MAHA is discussed further in the answer to Data Interpretation question 3.6.

4.17

Accepted answer

Preretinal haemorrhage

The shape of an intraocular haemorrhage depends on its site. Preretinal bleeding occurs into a large potential space allowing blood to spread widely, often with a fluid level. Nerve fibre-layer haemorrhages are flame-shaped and obscure the retinal vessels. Intraretinal haemorrhages are confined by the retina as dots, deep to the vessels. Subretinal vessels can spread into a large space but are deep to the vessels. Finally, subchoroidal bleeds are large but appear grey due to overlying pigment.

4.18

Accepted answers

(a) Caseating granuloma

(b) Sarcoidosis (lupus pernio)
     Lupus vulgaris

The section shows a classical giant cell granuloma. Granulomatous lesions involving the face are restricted to sarcoidosis, tuberculosis, syphilis, Wegener's granulomatosis and foreign bodies.

> **Nose lesions**
> - Lupus pernio (sarcoidosis)
> - Lupus vulgaris (tuberculosis)
> - Lupus erythematosus (SLE)
> - Lepromatous leprosy (ENL or LL)
> - Leishmaniasis (cutaneous or PKDL)
> - Acne rosacea
>
> - Rhinophyma
> - Nasal diphtheria (perinasal crusting)
> - Collapsed nasal cartilage
>   Wegener's granulomatosis
>   Syphilis
>   Lepromatous leprosy
>   Relapsing polychondritis

4.19

Accepted answers

Multiple hepatic metastases
Multifocal primary hepatoma

The most common multiple liver lesions, hyper- or hypoechoic on ultrasound, are metastases. Multifocal primary liver cancer can appear similar. Abscesses appear hypoechoic, i.e. dark.

4.20

Accepted answers

(a) Periarticular osteoporosis
     Periarticular erosions
     Loss of joint space
     Relative sparing of terminal interphalangeal joints
     Erosion of ulnar styloid
     Loss of carpal architecture
     Subluxation, most marked at the metacarpophalangeal joint of the thumb

(b) Rheumatoid arthritis

Knowledge of the sequence of events in rheumatoid allows early radiological diagnosis:
- Synovial inflammation shows as soft tissue swelling.
- Hyperaemia and disease leads to periarticular osteoporosis.
- Destruction of cartilage causes loss of joint space.
- Destruction of bone at the margins of synovial pannus results in erosions.
- Finally, subluxation and deformity give way to fibrosis and ankylosis.

Answers to Pictorial Material Paper 5

5.1

Accepted answer

Iron deficiency anaemia

Rejected answers

Multiple myeloma
Liver disease
Sideroblastic anaemia

The red cells show microcytosis and hypo-chromasia. The commonest cause for this anaemia is iron deficiency.

5.2

Accepted answers

Ringworm
Tinea corporis
Annular erythema

Rejected answer

Erythema multiforme

These lesions show the classical lesions with well-defined margins which can occur any-where in the body.

5.3

Accepted answer

Right-sided aortic arch

The aortic 'knuckle' and descending aorta can be seen on the right side.

5.4

Accepted answers

Xanthomata (100%)
Hyperlipidaemia (100%)

See fuller discussion of hyperlipidaemia in the answer to Data Interpretation question 7.7. The clinical classification of xanthomata appears on the next page.

Type of xanthoma	Site	Associated hyperlipidaemia
Xanthelasma	Around eyes	None or type II
Tuberous xanthoma	Yellow papules on pressure points (e.g. knees and elbows)	Types II, III and secondary
Tendinous xanthoma	Fingers and Achilles tendon	Types II, III and secondary
Eruptive xanthoma	Multiple lesions on buttocks/shoulders	Types II, III, IV, V and secondary (esp. diabetes)
Planar xanthoma	Palmar crease Macules at any site	Type II, III and secondary

5.5

Accepted answers

Chronic myeloid leukaemia (100%)
CML (50%)

Rejected answers

Multiple myeloma
Leukaemoid reaction

The blood film shows a complete spectrum of myeloid cells, with a few blasts. The levels of neutrophils and myelocytes exceeds those of blast cells and promyelocytes. The presence of splenomegaly helps distinguish CML from a severe leukaemoid reaction in marrow infiltration.

5.6

Accepted answers

(a) Nodules on chest wall

(b) Cysticercosis
Paragonamiasis

Subcutaneous nodules are seen on the chest wall. The patient has eosinophilia and a history of fits. This is in keeping with a diagnosis of cysticercosis. Paragonamiasis can also sometimes present with subcutaneous (and indeed brain) cysts.

5.7

Accepted answers

(a) Peutz–Jegher syndrome

(b) Massive GI haemorrhage
Malignant change of gastric or duodenal polyps

(c) Autosomal dominant

Rejected answer

Hereditary haemorrhagic telangiectasia

Peutz–Jegher syndrome is transmitted as an autosomal dominant trait. It comprises intestinal polyposis and freckles on the lips, oral mucosa and elsewhere. There may be massive GI haemorrhage and the polyps may become malignant.

Faces and gastrointestinal disease

- Jaundice/spider naevi/parotids
    Liver disease
- Pigmentation of lips and oral mucosa
    Peutz–Jegher syndrome (polyps)
    Addison's disease (anorexia, nausea, vomiting, diarrhoea)
- Telangiectasia
    Hereditary haemorrhagic telangiectasia (gut bleeding)
    Scleroderma (dysphagia)

- White hair and lemon tinge
    Pernicious anaemia (hypochlorhydria)
- Exophthalmos, stare, lid retraction
    Thyrotoxicosis (diarrhoea)
- Coarse facial features, sparse hair, etc.
    Hypothyroid facies (constipation)
- Heliotrope rash
    Dermatomyositis (dysphagia, carcinoma)

5.8

Accepted answers

Psoriasis
Muscle wasting

As in clinical practice, psoriasis may be an incidental finding in the examination, both in this section and the clinical examination.

The essential descriptions of classical psoriatic plaques are:

- Non-itchy.
- Well circumscribed.
- Slightly raised.
- Silvery scales on a red background.
- Extensor surfaces, sacrum, scalp and genitalia affected.

Other features include:

- Nail changes.
- Arthropathy.

The differential diagnosis for muscle wasting is wide, the most important causes in Membership being nerve disease such as motor neurone disease (fasiculation, upper motor neurone signs and bulbar involvement) and peripheral neuropathy – a particular favourite being diabetic amyotrophy, which is essentially a mononeuropathy of the femoral nerve giving wasting of the quadriceps. In everyday practice, the most common cause is probably disuse in arthritides, trauma and prolonged illness. Myopathies do not cause muscle wasting.

5.9

Accepted answer

Anterior communicating artery aneurysm

If you are shown cerebral anteriograms, then you will most likely be shown an aneurysm. The trick is to know your anatomy and get the location right! This has to be an anterior communicating artery aneurysm because it is in the mid-line on the antero-posterior view of a carotid arterogram.

Thirty per cent of aneurysms are anterior communicating artery aneurysms, 25% are posterior communicating aneurysms and 20% arise at the middle cerebral bifurcation. Twenty per cent of aneurysms are multiple. Posterior communicating aneurysms are associated with third nerve palsies.

5.10

Accepted answers

(a) Tick bite eschar

(b) Trypanosomal chancre
    Trypanosomiasis
    Tick typhus
    African tick typhus
    Rickettsial infection

Causes of eschars	
Anthrax	Trypansomal chancre
Orf	Burns
Tick typhus	Snake bite

5.11

Accepted answers

(a) Koilonychia
    Conjunctival pallor

(b) Hookworm-induced iron deficiency anaemia

Rejected answer

Iron deficiency anaemia

In addition to pallor and koilonychia the signs of iron deficiency anaemia include stomatitis, tongue papillary atrophy, glossitis, nail changes (thin, brittle, lacklustre nails, longitudinal ridging and flattening). Mild splenomegaly may be found. Blood film in iron deficiency anaemia shows a microcytic hypochromic picture with anisocytosis and poikilocytosis. Severe anaemia may lead to breathlessness and cardiac failure. Hookworm infection (usually *Ankylostoma duodenale* or *Necator americanus*) are the most common causes of iron deficiency anaemia in the tropics.

5.12

Accepted answers

Plasmodium falciparum malaria (100%)

Malaria (50%)

The peripheral blood film shows red blood cells infested with ring trophozoites. The presence of two rings in a single cell, or heavy parasitaemia as in this case, indicates falciparum malaria.

5.13

Accepted answers	*Rejected answer*
(a) Oesophageal varices	Oesophageal *Candida*

(b) Liver cirrhosis
  Portal pipe stem fibrosis
  Budd–Chiari syndrome
  Obstruction of the extrahepatic portal
    vein

Large cobblestone defects with a smooth outline in parts of the oesophagus suggests varices. Obviously in the clinical setting the history is extremely helpful in making the diagnosis. Varices are often confused with candidiasis by examination candidates. Oesophageal candidiasis on barium swallow is seen as a diffuse, small cobblestone outline of the whole of the barium filled oesophagus. Carcinoma shows up as an irregular narrowing in part of the oesophagus. Compare with Pictorial Material question 2.12.

5.14

Accepted answers

(a) Rubeosis iridis
  Neovascularization of the iris

(b) Diabetes mellitus

For discussion of diabetic eye disease, see answer to Pictorial Material question 1.13.

5.15

Accepted answers

(a) Red blood cell agglutination

(b) The Donarth–Landsteiner antibody

(c) Paroxysmal cold haemoglobinuria

This is a rare condition which used to arise following congenital syphilis, but now occurs following viral infections such as mumps, measles and chickenpox. The condition can also develop spontaneously with recurrent attacks over many years. Acute intravascular haemolysis occurs on exposure to cold, resulting in abdominal pain, Raynaud's phenomenon, peripheral cyanosis, haemoglobinuria, haemoglobinaemia and possibly a transient leukopenia. The recurrent form occurs mainly in adult males and the acute form in children. Cold agglutinins also occur in lymphoma and mycoplasma infection.

5.16

Accepted answers

Malignant stricture (100%)
Carcinoma of the oesophagus (100%)

Stricture of the oesophagus (25%)

The narrowing of the lumen with irregularity and shouldering of the mucosal outline suggests a malignant stricture. Benign strictures usually have a smooth mucosal outline and no 'shouldering'.

5.17

Accepted answer

Multiple myeloma (myelomatosis)

The bone marrow shows an increased number of plasma cells (>10%), many with abnormal forms. The peripheral blood film often shows marked rouleaux formation, and contains occasional plasma cells in about 15% of cases.

5.18

Accepted answers

(a) Rose spot

(b) Blood culture
       Bone marrow culture
       Stool culture
       Widal test

Rose spots (distinct discrete pinkish macules or maculopapules) are typical of typhoid fever and may appear towards the end of the first week up to the twentieth day. They occur in 50% of adults with typhoid and less frequently in children. The rash is distributed over the abdomen, chest and back. The College might be fussy about stool cultures in constipated patients!

5.19

Accepted answers

(a) Bamboo spine
  Intervertebral calcification

(b) Ankylosing spondylitis

Pattern recognition again.

5.20

Accepted answers

Hard exudates
Dot haemorrhage/microaneurysm

This is background diabetic retinopathy; the significant changes are well lateral to the macula. See answer to Pictorial Material question 1.13.

APPENDIX A – NORMAL RANGES

There are a few very basic investigations for which you will not be provided normal ranges in the MRCP examination. You will have to memorize these in advance if you have not already absorbed them by osmosis. We think the following lists include the only cases in which this will apply.

Haematology

	Male adult	Female adult
Hb (g/dl)	13.3–17.7	11.7–15.7
MCV (fl)	80.5–99.7	80.8–100.0
MCH (pg)	26.6–33.8	26.4–34.1
MCHC (g/dl)	31.5–36.3	32.4–35.8
WBC ($\times 10^9$/l)	3.9–10.6	3.5–11.0
Platelets ($\times 10^9$/l)	150–440	150–440

	Percentage	Absolute count
Neutrophils ($\times 10^9$/l)	40–75	1.8–7.7
Eosinophils ($\times 10^9$/l)	1–6	0–0.45
Basophils ($\times 10^9$/l)	0–1	0–0.20
Monocytes ($\times 10^9$/l)	0–8	0–0.8
Lymphocytes ($\times 10^9$/l)	20–45	1.0–4.8

ESR (age <60 y)   <15 mm in first hour

Biochemistry

Plasma sodium	135–145 mmol/l
Plasma potassium	3.5–5.0 mmol/l
Plasma urea	2.5–6.7 mmol/l
Plasma creatinine	70–150 μmol/l
Plasma bicarbonate	24–30 mmol/l
Plasma chloride	95–105 mmol/l
Plasma albumin	35–50 g/l
Plasma total protein	60–80 g/l
Plasma glucose (fasting)	4.0–6.0 mmol/l
Plasma bilirubin	3–17 μmol/l
Plasma calcium (total)	2.12–2.65 mmol/l
Plasma phosphate (inorganic)/inorganic phosphorus	0.8–1.45 mmol/l

Arterial blood gases

pH	7.38–7.44 kPa
$PaCO_2$	4.7–6.0 kPa
PaO_2	12.0–14.5 kPa

Cerebrospinal fluid analysis

Opening pressure	50–150 mm H_2O
Protein	0.15–0.40 g/l
Glucose	3.3–4.4 mmol/l

APPENDIX B – APPROACH TO A 12 LEAD ECG
IN THE MRCP PART 2
WRITTEN PAPER

Checklist

- Sensitivity marker
- Rate
- Mean Frontal Axis
- P wave
    height
    width
    shape
    relationship to QRS complexes
- PR interval
    length
    consistency
- Rhythm
    origin
    activation sequence
- QRS complex
    Q waves
    height/depth of QRS
    width of QRS
    pattern
- QT interval
- ST segments
    displacement
    gradient
    morphology
- T waves
    inverted or upright
    morphology

Sensitivity marker

Convention: The standard sensitivity marker (1 mV) measures 10 mm at full sensitivity, and 5 mm at half sensitivity. It may have been necessary to set the ECG machine at half sensitivity to fit in particularly large QRS complexes, e.g. in left ventricular hypertrophy. All the figures provided in this appendix assume that the ECG machine has been calibrated at standard sensitivity and speed.

Rate

Normal range: 55–100/min.

Mean Frontal Axis

Normal range: −30° to +90°.

Calculating the mean frontal axis, usually referred to simply as 'the axis', has been endowed with much mystery and needless misery. The underlying idea is simple: that the heart is assessed in a single two-dimensional coronal plan. An analogy might help: imagine you are looking down on an area of land from an aeroplane. You will only see movements in two dimensions. If there were a hot air balloon coming straight up it would not appear to be moving until it got close, and even then you would only assume it was moving from the fact that it appeared to be getting bigger. In terms of your two-dimensional plane, it would not be moving at all.

The mean frontal axis is the sum of all the movements of the wave of depolarization in that two-dimensional coronal plane over the whole period of depolarization. Let us go back to the aeroplane: imagine that a group of people are standing in the top left-hand corner of a field and over a few minutes they drift towards the bottom right-hand corner (figure 1a). You are too far away to be able to count every movement and add them up, but you can get a general impression that the movements are happening rapidly and simultaneously. Figure 1b represents the sum of the movements of these individuals; by analogy, the ECG represents the sum of the 'electrical movements'.

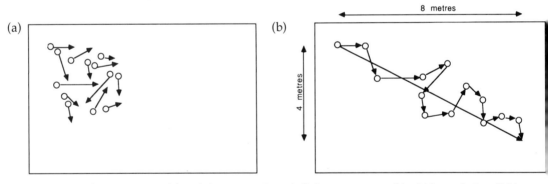

Figure 1   The movements (a) and the summation of all the movements (b) of 13 people in a field.

In an ECG, this 'sum of the electrical movements' is assessed by measuring the amplitudes of the QRS complexes in the limb leads. Standard lead I has an orientation of left to right (by convention labelled 0°; figure 2). It is the equivalent of looking at our field from its north side. In one dimensional terms, the total movement of our group of people with respect to the north side of the field is 8 metres. Standard lead aVF has the orientation north to south (by convention labelled 90°; figure 2). It is the equivalent of looking at our field from its west side. In one dimensional terms, the total movement of our group of people with respect to the west side of the field is 4 metres. These two vectors can be added together nose to tail to estimate the direction of the mass movement (figure 3).

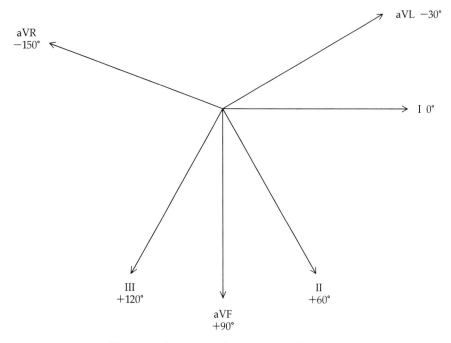

Figure 2   Conventional orientation of limb leads.

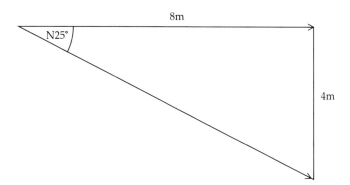

Figure 3   Resultant vector of movements in figure 1.

Using the extent of deflection of the ECG as a measure of movement of the wave of depolarization and repolarization, an identical process can be performed to calculate the mean frontal axis.
However, the precision of measurement of the deflection is such that it is meaningless to report
the angle to less than the nearest 5°.

Here are two worked examples:

Example 1:

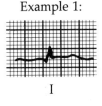

I

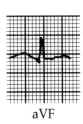

aVF

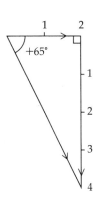

Example 1

(1) In lead I, the net sum of forces in the QRS complex is +2 mm (3 mm positive deflection from which subtract 1 mm negative deflection).
(2) In lead aVF, it is +4 mm (5 mm positive, 1 mm negative).
(3) Add the vectors of these two leads together in a nose-to-tail manner; both are positive, thus they are oriented in the direction of the lead.
(4) The mean frontal axis is the resultant vector, approximately +65°. This is normal.

Example 2:

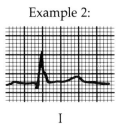

I

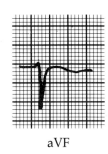

aVF

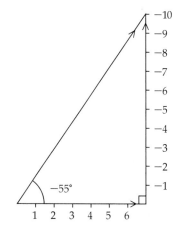

Example 2

(1) In lead I, the net sum of forces is +7 mm (8 mm positive deflection, 1 mm negative deflection).
(2) In lead aVF, it is −10 mm (1 mm positive, and 11 mm negative).
(3) Add these vectors nose-to-tail, taking into account the fact that aVF is negative, and thus goes away from the direction of the normal vector of aVF (i.e. −90° rather than +90°).
(4) The mean frontal axis is thus approximately −55°. This is left axis deviation.

In a short period of time, you should be able to calculate axes in your head. For most clinical purposes, it is enough to be no more precise than ±30°. The only real exception to this is when you are trying to compare the QRS axis with the T axis.

Some rules of thumb

- If the complexes in I and II are both predominantly positive, the axis is normal.
- The axis lies at 90° to an isoelectric complex, i.e. positive and negative deflections are equal in size.

Note: While it is usually effective to use leads I and aVF to calculate the mean frontal axis, occasionally it seems that all leads seem to have an isoelectric complex and no axis can be calculated. This is presumably because the true axis is nearly perpendicular to the coronal plane.

P wave

Normal dimentions: Height: 0.25 mV (0.5 mm)
                                          Width: 0.12 s (3 mm)

Leads to view: the lead with the large P waves should be used. Leads II and V1 are usually the best.

(1) *Height:* P waves more than 0.25 mV tall (2.5 mm) in the limb leads imply right atrial enlargement.
(2) *Width:* P waves more than 0.12 s wide (3 mm) in the limb leads imply left atrial enlargement.
(3) *Shape:* in right atrial enlargement, the P waves are tall, in left atrial enlargement, they are broad and bifid. Also in left atrial enlargement, in V1 the P wave is biphasic with a negative component that is at least one small square in area and larger than the area of the positive component.
   If the P waves look unusual, e.g. prominent in leads in which they are usually poorly seen, or predominantly negative, they may not be originating from the sinus node. They may be ectopic within the atria, or be originating from the atrio-ventricular node or junction and be being retrogradely conducted. In the latter case, they tend to be predominantly negative. Alternatively, they may in fact be the F or f waves of atrial flutter or fibrillation respectively. Suspect atrial flutter if the rate is ventricular rate is approximately 150/min (i.e. 2:1 AV block: the atrial rate is 300/min). Suspect atrial fibrillation if the ventricular rhythm is irregular.
   Note for the perverse: beloved of examiners is the ECG in which the baseline clearly looks like atrial fibrillation but the ventricular rate is strictly regular. The catch is that there is also complete heart block. There are therefore two independent foci of electrical activation: the fibrillating atria and the isolated ventricles.
(4) *Relationship with QRS complexes:* the presence of true P waves implies sinus rhythm. Check that each is followed by a QRS complex. If not, then there is at least second degree heart block.

PR interval

The PR interval stretches from the *beginning* of the P wave to the *beginning* of the QRS complex.

Normal range: 0.12 –0.20 s (3–5 mm).

Leads to view: use the lead in which the P wave is best seen (usually II and V1) and accept the longest measurement of the PR interval.

(1) *Length:* if it is longer than 0.02 s, there is some degree of heart block. If it is shorter than 0.12 s, this implies either (a) that there is an accessory pathway with rapid conduction between the atria and ventricles (Wolff–Parkinson–White, Lown–Ganong–Levine syndrome, etc.) or (b) that the P wave is not originating from the sinu-atrial node. Atrial ectopic foci may be associated with a short PR interval, as are beats originating from the AVN. If the pacemaker is distal in the junctional tissue, the wavefront may depolarize the ventricles before the atria, in which case there is a consistent relationship between the QRS complex and a P wave which is seen *after* it. In the intermediate situation of a pacemaker in the centre of the junctional tissue, P wave and QRS complex coincide and the former may not be seen.

(2) *Consistency:* make sure the relationship between P waves and QRS complex is seen in all, or nearly all, leads. If the relationship is not consistent, consider second or third degree heart block.

Rhythm

The term rhythm, refers to two things: (1) the origin of the wave of depolarization and (2) the sequence in which it proceeds, the 'activation sequence'. You have gathered all the necessary information to determine both by examining the P waves and the PR interval.

(1) *The origin of the wave of depolarization:* in normal rhythm the sequence begins at the sinu-atrial node, producing sinus rhythm. However, it may begin anywhere else in the heart. Other sources within the conduction system include the atrio-ventricular node (AVN). It is this 'node' which is referred to in the term 'nodal rhythm'. The term 'junctional rhythm' is less anatomically specific and implies a rhythm originating from the junction of the atria and ventricles. This includes the AVN and also the specialized conduction tissue distal to it, the bundle of His. If the sequence is triggered from a point anywhere else in the myocardium, it is an ectopic rhythm. These may take over control of cardiac depolarization for a single beat, a run, or for prolonged periods, and may be atrial or ventricular. Any such non-sinus supraventricular origin of the rhythm may produce an atypical P wave, which in turn may be conducted anterogradely and/or retrogradely.

In certain circumstances, there is continuous electrical activity in parts of the heart, most commonly *atrial flutter* and *fibrillation*. When these exist, they stimulate depolarization of the ventricles and are the origin of the activation sequence.

Finally, it is possible to have more than one source of depolarization operating at the same time. Most commonly, one or more ectopic foci and the sinu-atrial node are firing simultaneously. Which is responsible for a particular cardiac beat depends entirely on the timing of each with respect to adjacent refractory periods, and the source may change from moment to moment. Occasionally, they share responsibility for a single beat, with their respective waves of depolarization meeting half-way. This is the origin of the fusion beat. In complete heart block, the atria and ventricles are electrically isolated from each other and each has a separate source of depolarization.

(2) *The activation sequence:* in normal beats the wave of depolarization originating in the sinu-atrial node passes through the atria to the AVN, bundle of His, the specialized conducting tissue in the ventricles and from these through the ventricular myocardium. This can be interrupted or slowed at any point. If there is a delay or blockage in the area of the AVN or

bundle of His, then this is a form of heart block. More distal blocks may produce left and right bundle branch blocks and hemiblocks.

QRS complex

Examine all QRS complexes in sequence. Bear in mind the sequence of orientation (figure 2). We suggest looking at the limb leads first in the order: aVL, I, II, aVF, III, and aVR and then at the chest leads in order V1–V6. Consider each of the following points:

(1) *Are there any Q waves and are they pathological?* Q waves may be found in any lead of a normal ECG except V2. To be pathological, however, they must be at least 0.04 s in duration (one small square) and in the vertical axis be more than 25% of the height of the ensuing R wave. Even then, what appears to be a pathological Q wave may actually be a prominent S wave which has completely obliterated the R wave. Since it is then the first deflection of the QRS complex and is negative it conforms to the definition of a Q wave. These waves are called QS waves and may be seen in aVL, III and V1. A QS wave (or apparently pathological Q wave) is normal in aVL if the axis is $> +60°$ and normal in III if the axis is $< +30°$.

(2) *The height/depth of QRS complexes:* at least one R wave in the precordial leads must be greater than 8 mm. Otherwise, the QRS complexes may be said to be pathologically small. The definition of pathologically tall/deep QRS complexes is complex. The size of the R wave in aVL must not exceed 13 mm and in aVF, 20 mm. In the chest leads, the tallest R wave should not exceed 27 mm and the deepest S/QS wave should not exceed 30 mm. The sum of the tallest R wave and the deepest S/QS should not exceed 40 mm. If any of these dimensions is exceeded, the ECG cannot be declared unequivocally normal. However, it is harder to assert that a particular chamber is hypertrophied without accompanying ST/T wave abnormalities, particularly in young people.

(3) *The width of QRS complexes:* no QRS complex should exceed 0.12 s (three small squares). If it does, this implies an intraventricular conduction defect. This may be due to ventricular hypertrophy or a defect in the conduction system. Look at the height of the complexes and their morphology for further clues.

(4) *Pattern:* normally, R waves become progressively taller across the chest, but it is a normal variant for them to decrease in size from V4 to V5. Conversely, S waves should become progressively smaller across the chest, although V1 may be smaller than V2. Finally, the morphology of broadened complexes may characterize a pattern of conduction defects.

QT interval

Prolonged QT intervals may be due to metabolic abnormalities (e.g. hypocalcaemia) or drugs (e.g. amiodarone, quinidine, disopyimide), or be a congenital abnormality (e.g. Romano–Ward syndrome). It may be associated with significant dysrhythmias, but it is difficult to assess since it is rate related. (So is the PR-interval, but it varies rather less.) The QT interval may be corrected using the formula $QTc = QT/\sqrt{(R-R)}$. This produces the range of 0.35–0.43 s. However, rather than calculate this on each occasion, some find it easier to note a few specific values:

Rate (per min)	Upper limit of QT interval (seconds) Male	Female
150	0.25	0.28
100	0.31	0.34
75	0.36	0.39
60	0.40	0.44
50	0.44	0.48

ST segments

The ST segment runs from the J point, the *end* of the S wave, to the *beginning* of the T wave.

(1) *Displacement from the isoelectric line:* the ST segment must not deviate from the isoelectric line by more than 1 mm either upwards or downwards. However, it often slopes, causing much angst in quantifying the degree of deviation. In exercise ECG testing, the crucial place at which deviation is assessed is taken to be 0.06 s (1.5 small squares) along the ST segment from the J point.

(2) *Gradient:* a downsloping ST segment is much more likely to imply significant ischaemic heart disease than an upsloping one, even if both are 1 mm depressed 0.06 s from the J point. However, it can only finally be interpreted in the light of the clinical scenario.

(3) *Morphology:* pericarditis is associated with saddle-shaped ST elevation in many leads of the ECG. Some apparent ST elevation is often shrugged off as an abnormally 'high take-off' and of no clinical significance, and may be a normal racial variant. This is usually seen in the right precordial leads. It can be difficult to assert what is significant ST segment elevation in leads V1–V3. Again, the apparent abnormality must be interpreted in the clinical context, and mild to moderate (<2 mm) ST elevation in V1–V3 with no other ECG abnormality is unlikely to be significant unless accompanied by clinical features of right ventricular infarction.

T waves

(1) *Inverted or upright:* inverted T waves can only be said to be unequivocally abnormal if they are found in I, II, or V4–V6. They may or may not be pathological if found in other leads. Of more value is the assertion that a T wave should be upright if the QRS complex in that lead is predominantly positive, and inverted if the QRS is predominantly negative. There can be a small amount of deviation from this rule, but almost never in more than one lead. The T wave axis (calculated in the same way as the QRS axis) should not differ from the mean frontal axis by more than 45°. The one exception to this rule is in inferior infarction, when inverted T waves are abnormal findings (part of the ECG findings of MI) despite having a similar axis to the QRS complexes.

(2) *Morphology:* peaked or flattened T waves are found in metabolic abnormalities, e.g. peaked in hyperkalaemia and flattened (with ensuing U waves) in hypokalaemia. Size should be assessed in leads V3–V6. The T wave should be no more than $\frac{2}{3}$ and no less than $\frac{1}{8}$ of the height of the preceding R wave.

INDEX OF LISTS

INDEX